Bronwyn Whitlocke, a Shiatsu Therapist and Chinese Medicine Herbalist and Acupuncturist has twenty years of professional and practical experience. Bronwyn believes that health can be achieved using natural and non-intrusive remedies. Her common sense approach encourages individuals to understand and maintain their own health.

Acknowledgements

This book is dedicated to my clients; they were the inspiration for this book.

I also want to thank particularly Patricia Sharp, Sheila Hill, Jo Hafey, Hetty Veldman and Caroline Baum for their support and positive criticisms in achieving an easily understood book.

How To Use This Book

I want this book to be a useful tool in helping you to understand your own body. Therefore, the book can be read from beginning to end. Alternatively it can be used, just as effectively, by referring to a specific condition or area of concern.

Bronwyn Whitlocke

Chinese Medicine For Women

A Common sense Approach

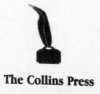

The Collins Press

This edition published by The Collins Press,
West Link Park, Doughcloyne, Wilton, Cork, 1999
Originally published by Spinifex Press, Australia, 1997

Edited by Janet Mackenzie
Indexed by Max McMaster
Text design and typesetting in ITC Garamond
and Tekton by Lynne Hamilton
Cover design by Ray Jalil: WHL Digital
Made and printed in Australia by Australian Print Group

A CIP catalogue for this book is available from the British Library

ISBN: 1-898256-61-6

For my mum, Amelia and daughter, Jessica, for their unfailing love and support.

CONTENTS

Introduction

This book is designed to be used as a quick guide for women in understanding their own bodies in terms of Traditional Chinese Medicine (TCM). In this book I look simply at the main meridians affecting the concerns and conditions of women's health. Most of the areas I cover have been recorded in both my professional and personal experiences; because many of my clients have asked how they can take charge of their own health, I have been prompted to write this book. I deal mainly with diet, lifestyle, menstruation, pregnancy and menopause. There are many good books that cover aspects of TCM in detail (recommended reading is listed in Appendix 5). This book will introduce you to the central concepts of TCM and areas of theory relevant to women's health.

My personal belief is that a practitioner should do three things: facilitate an understanding of why problems occur, get the body functioning, and help the client to understand her lifestyle and the changes she can make to minimise further problems. I would like to see women take responsibility for their health and be their own practitioners. In my opinion, TCM is the best way to do this, through lifestyle changes including

diet and exercise and less dependency on other practitioners. This does not mean that you ignore the signals
your body gives and keep away from any professional;
but you should know what to do for simple ailments,
not allowing them to fester into complicated problems
requiring long-term treatment.

This book is intended as an aid to an alternative
form of health practice; it is not seen as the only
source of help. TCM can give us a better understanding of our bodies in relation to our environment. TCM
can help and support treatment from others and is
not necessarily a modality that has to be used singly. It
works well with other health practices. It is a simple,
effective method with discernible results and does not
require a strong understanding of the theory of
Chinese Medicine to be implemented. My personal
belief is that TCM is a supportive therapy that can be
used in conjunction with other treatments. I would
like to see an embracing of it within the Western medical framework in mutual respect for the qualities of
each form of medicine.

Chinese medicine can support vigorous treatments
needed in some conditions and may help alleviate some
of the untoward side-effects of drugs and other aggres-
sive (although sometimes necessary) treatments.

The language in this book is specifically non-med-
ical, and Chinese terminology is kept to minimum. I
endeavour to present the information in simple English
to communicate to the lay person the benefits of TCM.

An Outline of Traditional Chinese Medicine

Chinese medicine can be traced through myth and legend back to the Shang Dynasty of 1766–1122 BC. One thousand years later, the concepts of Yin and Yang and the five elements arrived. Through the use of case histories, astute observation, and reflection on the nature of the world, Chinese medicine slowly evolved to become the science that it is today. In the twentieth century it was pushed aside for the new Western medicine through Japanese, American and European influences. Eventually, however, the need for basic health for the peasant population outside the cities prompted the Chinese leaders at the time to create "barefoot doctors". These barefoot doctors used basic Western medicine, together with traditional Chinese medical practices of acupuncture, herbs, massage and diet, to help the people in poor and remote communities.

TCM is a unique system that looks at the human body in terms of its environment. It looks at the nature of things. What is the nature of the environment, food, and our emotions? TCM talks of dampness, cold, heat and wind as one would talk of the environment and its effects. For example, in our environment, heat causes fluids to dry up; excessive heat can even crack the earth; heat can make one feel lethargic or slow. Similarly, heat in the body shows as a dry, sometimes cracked, tongue, thirst, a feeling of heat (usually in the head, as heat rises), redness, swelling, headache (inability of heat to escape), lack of energy, and the pulse may be rapid.

To explain these phenomena, Traditional Chinese Medicine has its own terms. The most common are Qi, Yin and Yang, together with Blood, fluids and meridians. The following explanations are simplified to provide a basic understanding of the theory of TCM.

Yin and Yang

Simply, Yin and Yang are two polar complements. They are a convenient form to describe functions of change within the universe, whether the universe be external (environment) or internal (body). Classically, Yin and Yang can be divided as shown in Table 1.

Table 1
Characteristics associated with Yin and Yang

Yin	Yang
Internal	External
Cold	Hot
Contracting	Expanding
Watery	Dry
Heavy	Light
Chronic	Acute
Deficiency	Excess
Female	Male
Generation of Blood	Metabolism

Blood is internal and specifically Yin. Women are perceived as Yin because of the association with blood in menstruation and pregnancy. Fluids (Jin Ye) are also associated with Yin. Fluids include internal fluids, urine and perspiration.

The main meridians (see page 6) associated with menstruation and reproduction are Spleen, Liver and Kidney, all Yin meridians. Yin meridians are so called because they occur on the inside aspect of the body, and therefore have a strong connection with blood production, blood storage, and reproduction. In contrast, Yang meridians occur on the outer aspect of the body and deal with metabolic activity and protection of the body.

TCM looks at aspects of Yin and Yang and it is the basis of this medicine to identify over-abundance or decline of either Yin or Yang. Referring to Table 1, if there is a chronic condition that has gone on for a long time and become internal, affecting not only the external body but also the deeper areas of meridians and organs, we can see that there may be a Yang deficiency leading to a predominance of Yin. A healthy individual will have a balance of Yin and Yang. In Figure 1, showing the classical representation of Yin and Yang, it can be seen that as Yin slowly reduces and becomes Yang; there is also a small amount of Yin in Yang and Yang in Yin. It is this continuous cycle that must be kept in harmony for health.

Qi

Qi (pronounced *chee*) is the life force or vital energy that flows through the meridians. All the Qi in the

Figure 1. The classical representation of Yin and Yang.

body is referred to in general terms as Normal or Upright Qi or True Qi. The Chinese refer to three sources of Normal Qi:

- prenatal Qi (Jing), transmitted to the child at conception and stored in the Kidneys
- grain or nutritive Qi which is derived from the digestion of food
- natural air Qi, extracted by the Lungs from the air we breathe.

Qi has five natural functions which we will examine in turn.

Movement

Qi is the source of all movement in the body: physical movement, involuntary muscular responses, mental functioning, growth and life processes. In the body, Qi is in constant movement, either ascending or descending, entering or leaving. Normal Qi activity is harmonious. If there is insufficient Qi, or it is obstructed or moves in rebellion or recklessly, or it loses its regulation, disharmony will result. If Qi is rebellious, it means that it is moving against its normal pattern. For instance, Lung Qi normally descends, pulling in air to feed the Lungs and support other metabolic functions;

when Lung Qi rebels, a cough or shortness of breath is a usual indicator. Obstructions of Qi (blockages in the flow of Qi) are usually indicated by a specific sort of pain that is relieved by pressure. In the condition of deficient Qi (where there is not enough Qi to flow through the meridians) there can be lethargy.

Protection

Qi resists pathological entry to the body (external pernicious influences). That is to say, there is a Protective Qi that protects the external parts of the body from invasions of infection, whether viral or bacterial, and also from invasions of Cold, Heat, Damp or Dryness. The common cold can sometimes be classified (depending on the symptoms) as a Wind Cold invasion or Wind Heat invasion. Wind Cold invasion is due to the external environment of Cold and Wind entering the body and affecting the natural internal equilibrium. Wind Heat invasion can be caused by an overheated environment such as an office. This overheating can produce sweating (abnormal in a cold climate) which weakens Protective Qi, allowing Heat to enter the body.

Harmonious Transformation

Qi transforms ingested food into other substances, such as Blood, other forms of Qi, and fluids such as tears, sweat and urine. Nutritive Qi is derived from the food we ingest. It passes through the stomach to the Spleen (this term has a different meaning to that of Western medicine; see Meridians, page 6). Spleen Qi further transforms Qi into a higher form, helping to support blood and fluid production. This process can be compared to the process of a still, where solid products are introduced into a boiling vat and the resulting product is a less solid but more "pure" essence. This is one reason why diet is seen as a major part of therapy and a support of preventive good health.

Retains Body's Substances and Organs

Qi keeps blood in the vessels, keeps organs in their place in the body, and prevents excessive loss of fluids. When the Spleen Qi is deficient, because its ability is to hold and push up, there may be prolapse of the bowel or uterus. If Heat is present in the blood, it will cause the blood to overflow the vessels, resulting in haemorrhage.

Warms the Body

The fifth function of Qi is to maintain normal body heat.

A TCM practitioner who talks about a disharmony of Qi may refer to a deficiency, a collapse, a stagnation or a rebellion.

Meridians

Meridians are channels through which Qi flows. There are Yin and Yang meridians of Spleen, Kidney, Liver, Lung, Small Intestine, Large Intestine, Heart, Gall Bladder, and Pericardium. They are so named because of close association with the organs, but the translation from Chinese to acceptable English forms sometimes shows no resemblance to the organ named. Along the paths of the meridian are points or "gates" which stimulate Qi in some form to calm, harmonise or build Qi. This can be done by a number of methods; the most common are:

- *Acupuncture*: Fine, hair-like needles are inserted into the points or "gates".
- *Cupping*: Cups are used to release stagnation; they are heated and attached to the skin surface by suction.
- *Moxabustion*: Localised heat is applied using either loose or compressed moxa, a herb known for its dispersing and warm nature (see Appendix 1).
- *Herbs*: Qi flow is adjusted internally through the ingestion of herbal soups or pills.
- *Shiatsu*: Points and meridians are stimulated by pressure with the fingers, thumbs or palms.
- *Exercise*: Programmes such as Qi Qong and Tai Chi facilitate the harmonious flow of Qi to support health and longevity.
- *Diet*: Particular foods support Qi flow, build blood and fluids, support body and mental function.

As we have seen, meridians are named after certain Western terms for organs, although the organ does not always correspond with the meridian it is named after. This means that, in the case of a problem with, say, the Liver meridian, there is not always a correlation with an organic problem of the organ called the Liver that is discernible to Western medicine. If you accept that the meridians have names similar to terms used in Western medicine but do not necessarily indicate a Western medical condition, understanding of TCM will flow more easily.

The following information will be better understood if it is interpreted through the Yin and Yang theory of transforming (changing) and circulating substances (see Table 2). The function of the meridians is to receive food and fluids taken from the external environment, and to change these into substances (Blood, Qi, Fluids) and waste products (urine, faeces). The meridians are also responsible for maintaining harmony within the body and its external environment by ensuring Qi is flowing unblocked around the body.

Table 2
Meridian pairs associated with Yin and Yang

Yin	Yang
Kidney	Bladder
Spleen	Stomach
Liver	Gall Bladder
Heart	Small Intestine
Lungs	Large Intestine
Pericardium	Triple Warmer

The Yin meridians are deep and internal. They are responsible for the creation, change, storage, release and regulation of pure substances: Qi, Blood, Jing, Fluids and Shen (described on pages 20–22). Yang meridians are superficial and external; they are responsible for receiving and storing food and drink, movement and absorption of the changed products, and excretion of wastes.

Therefore, in terms of TCM, there is a continuous

movement as in the Yin Yang theory of filling and emptying.

The following explanations first give the name of the system; which aspect of the body it governs; its functions and the substances it governs; its associated emotions; where the system reflects in the body; where it opens into the body; and any special relationships with other systems or substances.

Spleen, Stomach

Governs	Change and movement within the digestive system.
Substances	Nutritive Qi, Fluids, Blood.
Functions	• Governs movement and transformation (change) of food to substances.
	• Governs ascension—its natural movement is to pull up and hold. For instance Spleen Qi deficiency may indicate prolapse of bowel or uterus
	• Manages Blood by holding it in its vessels.
Emotions	Pensiveness, thoughtfulness, worry, compassion.
Reflects in	Flesh, muscles and four limbs.
Opens into	Mouth and lips.
Relationships	Liver (storage of blood) and Kidney Yang (warmth for digestive fire).

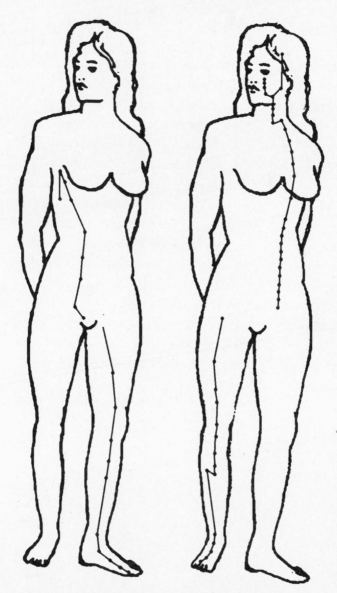

Figure 2. Left, the Spleen meridian;
right, the Stomach meridian.

Lung, Large Intestine

Governs	Respiration and the formation of Qi in Lungs.
Substances	Qi, Fluids, Protective Qi.
Functions	• Disperses and descends Qi and Fluids.
	• Regulates the upper water passages.
	• Regulates the surface body with Protective Qi which helps to prevent infection invading the body.
Emotions	Grief and communication.
Opens into	Nose.
Reflects in	Skin and body hair.
Relationships	Heart, Spleen, Kidney, Large Intestine—all need fluids for their appropriate functions.

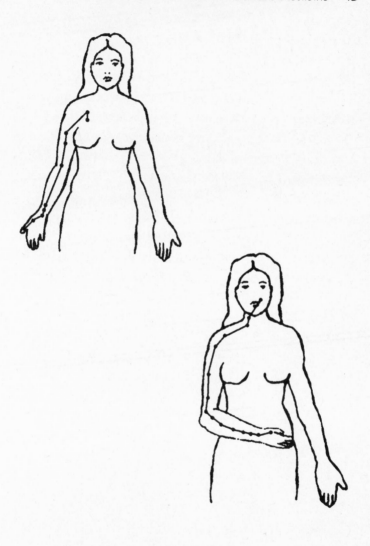

*Figure 3. Left, the Lung meridian;
right, the Large Intestine meridian.*

Heart, Small Intestine

Governs	Blood and Blood vessels.
Substances	Blood and Shen (Spirit or Mind).
Functions	• Controls Blood circulation.
	• Stores Shen.
Emotions	Joy, consciousness, self-awareness.
Opens into	Tongue.
Reflects in	The complexion of the face.
Relationships	Spleen for Blood. Small intestine and Kidney for Fluids balance.

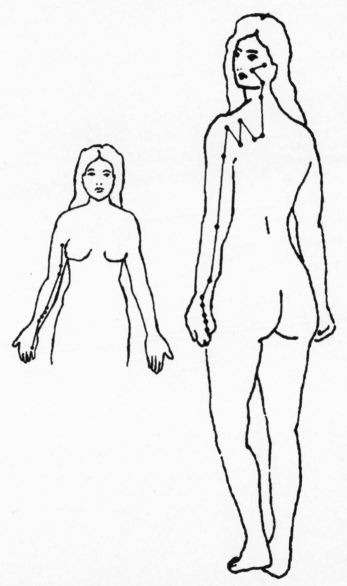

Figure 4. Left, the Heart meridian; right, the Small Intestine meridian.

Liver, Gall Bladder

Governs	Smooth flow of Qi and digestion.
Substances	Qi, bile, Blood.
Functions	• Controls free flow of Qi.
	• Controls tendons.
	• Stores Blood.
Emotions	Decision-making, anger, shouting, appropriate action.
Opens into	Eyes.
Reflects in	Nails and tendons.
Relationships	The eyes, Spleen (Blood), Gall Bladder (break-down of foods).

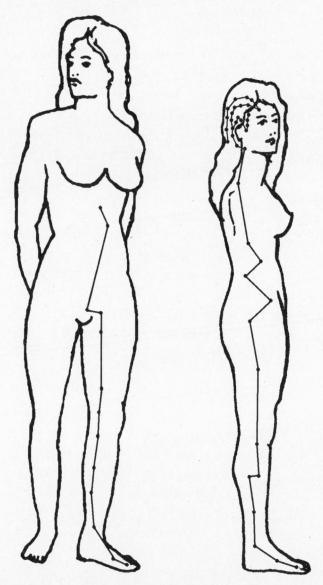

*Figure 5. Left, the Liver meridian;
right, the Gall Bladder meridian.*

Kidney, Bladder

Governs	Birth, growth, development, decline and death.
Substances	Qi, Jing, Fluids.
Functions	• Stores Jing.
	• Controls birth, growth, development, reproduction, death.
	• Controls bones and bone marrow.
	• Controls Fluids.
	• Kidney Yang controls opening and closing (sphincters).
Emotions	Fear, willpower.
Opens into	Ears, and sphincters of urethra and anus.
Reflected in	The head hair.
Relationships	Lung by grasping Lung Qi to allow respiration.

Pericardium and Triple Warmer

There is some controversy in regards to this pair of meridians because the names refer to no actual organ, as in the previous pairs, and it has no real form. Because of this, motion is attached to it, neither does it reflect into any body area. It is included because of its strong connection with the movement of body fluids and the balance of Qi throughout the body. There has been a misconception in the West that the Triple Warmer is associated with the endocrine system: this is not correct. Chinese medicine does not recognise this system and so there is now allowance within its medicine.

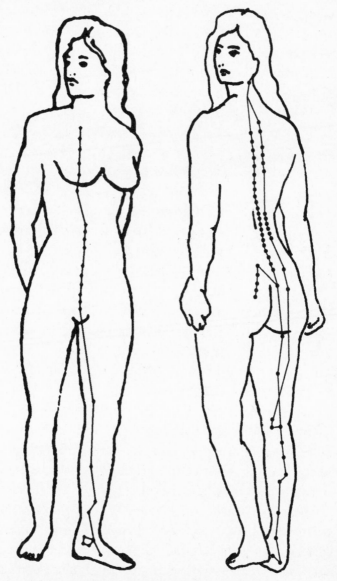

Figure 6. Left, the Kidney meridian;
right, the Bladder meridian.

Governs	Qi, Fluids; formation, transformation, circulation and excretion.
Substances	Body fluids, Qi.
Functions	Circulates and distributes Qi and Fluids to the organs.

The Triple Warmer has three metabolic levels:

Upper Burner	Distributes Qi through the body to warm and nourish the skin, muscles, tendons and bones; regulates skin and pores. The area it covers deals with the chest and abdominal cavity.
Middle Burner	Aids digestion. The area it covers deals with the Spleen and Stomach.
Lower Burner	Separates pure and impure essence and aids in the discharge of wastes (urine and faeces). The area it covers deals with the Kidney, Intestines and Bladder.

Blood

The TCM idea of Blood has some similarities with the Western conception of blood, but its characteristics and functions are not identical to Western functions.

The major activity of Blood is to circulate continuously, to nourish, maintain and moisten. Blood is a liquid and is considered a Yin substance. Blood originates through the transformation of food. The stomach ingests the food, and the Spleen "distills" it to a purified essence. The Spleen Qi transports this essence upward to the Lung, while Nutritive Qi turns the essence to Blood. Blood is pushed through the body by Heart Qi with Chest Qi. A TCM saying is: "Qi is the commander of the Blood, Blood is the mother of Qi."

Two major disharmonies of Blood are deficiency and stagnation. With deficient Blood, there is an insufficient nourishment of Blood to the body or a particular organ. Congealed or stagnant Blood is not flowing or is blocked; it usually relates to the Liver Qi. Conditions that may result from deficiency are anaemia, nervous exhaustion, hypotension (low blood pressure), and from stagnation, dysmenorrhea (painful periods) and other painful conditions.

Fluids

Fluids are liquids other than Blood. The function of the Fluids is to moisten and nourish the hair, skin, membranes, flesh, muscles, organs, joints, brain, marrow and bones. Fluids are derived from ingested food, and regulated by Lung and Kidney Qi and the kidneys.

Shen

Shen is the mind or spirit, and is housed in the Heart. Shen vitalises the body and consciousness, and provides the driving force behind the personality. It is reflected in the eyes.

Jing

Jing is inherited from the parents on conception. It is stored in the Kidneys and supports conception, growth and development. Jing cannot be renewed and slowly wanes as death nears. Jing is very precious, and to stop premature ageing it must be protected through a healthy lifestyle and diet.

The Five Phases or Elements

The Five Phases provide simple indicators for the lay person to see the movement of a condition and to trace it backwards to the root of the problem. The Five Phases refer to categories in the natural world, namely wood, earth, fire, metal and water.

These elements are seen to be indispensable for the maintenance of life and production, and they also represent five important states that initiate changes in the natural world. This is a simple concept to explain the effects that one condition can have on another. Although this explanation is simplistic, it can be of use in the clinical situation by supporting the diagnosis and treatment. This theory deals with movement and is a way to explain the effects of one organ on another, the emotions and the seasons affecting the whole person. Yin and Yang describe the interaction between sun and shade, heat and cold, dry and wet; in contrast, the Five Phases represent the seasons of the earth, the stages of human life, the waxing and waning of Yin and Yang.

The basis of Chinese medicine is that the forces that control the cycles of change in our world are duplicated in our bodies. Thus the Five Phases are an atlas of human cycles and change, charting the course of process. Human beings' cycles of life can be seen in the very similar cycles of nature—birth, growth, maturation and death.

The Water Phase is a time of gestation, a Yin time of internal and reflective qualities, waiting for spring. The Wood Phase is seen as birth or new life, a movement towards the Yang Peak, so spring is the season of fresh life and growth. The Fire Phase is the time of full growth, the peak of Yang. It moves on to the Earth Phase of maturation, where Yin starts to decline to the Metal Phase, leading finally to death.

Not only can the Five Phases indicate our life cycle but also the process of daily life. Figure 7 shows Yang peaking at midday and Yin at midnight. Qi moves through these aspects daily, affecting organs and meridians on a two-hourly basis (Figure 8). Stomach and Spleen are at their peak at 7 to 11 a.m., showing the need for a good breakfast while these organs are at their optimum. At 5 to 7 a.m. the Large Intestine peaks, indicating the natural rhythm of elimination. Most people find that this is the usual time (if regular) for a bowel movement. Symptoms of excess appear during peak hours, whereas deficiency shows up during ebb tides of Qi. Kidney Qi deficiency often appears at 5 to 7 a.m., with the early-morning need to urinate.

Table 3 shows associations of the Five Phases in regard to the emotions, climate, organs, orifices of the body, tissues of the body, and even smell or taste.

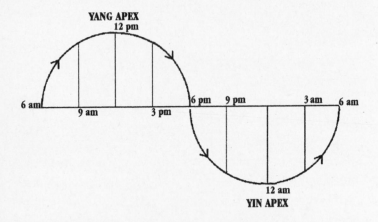

Figure 7. The daily cycles of Yin and Yang.

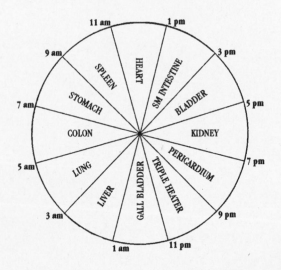

Figure 8. The daily movement of Qi.

Table 3
Attributes corresponding with the Five Phases

Attribute	Wood	Fire	Earth	Metal	Water
Season	spring	early summer	late summer	autumn	winter
Direction	east	south	centre	west	north
Colour	blue/ green	red	yellow	white	black
Climate	windy	hot	damp	dry	cold
Human sound	shouting	laughing	singing	weeping	groaning
Emotion	anger	joy	pensive- ness	grief	fear
Taste	sour	bitter	sweet	pungent	salty
Yin organ	Liver	Heart	Spleen	Lungs	Kidney
Yang organ	Gall Bladder	Small Intestine	Stomach	Large Intestine	Bladder
Orifice	eyes	tongue	mouth	nose	ears
Tissue	tendons	blood vessels	flesh	skin	bones
Smell	goatish	burning	fragrant	rank	rotten

The process of movement of the Five Phases can be shown metaphorically:

Water: nourishes Wood by moistening and restraining; it restrains Fire by quenching it.

Wood: generates Fire, and inhibits Earth.

Fire: generates Earth (ash to soil), and restrains Metal.

Earth: supports Metal, and controls Water.

Metal: vitalises Water, and restrains and inhibits Wood.

To use the Five Phases in a diagnosis, the practitioner asks about the emotions, unusual tastes in the mouth or cravings. For instance, in a consultation a client may complain of headaches, which can be caused by Heat, Liver Qi rebellion, or even Blood deficiency. To help differentiate, the practitioner uses some indicators from the Five Phases model to refine the diagnosis and so asks questions about attributes relating to Wood: sore or itchy eyes, anger, and possibly a sour taste in the mouth, as can be seen by referring to Table 3. If all the symptoms are experienced by the client, this might indicate that the Liver Qi requires some treatment.

This system is a useful tool for the lay person to understand the symptoms that are signals for some treatment to the affected area. So, if you have been experiencing some grief in your life that is affecting you strongly, you may also be experiencing uncontrolled weeping, maybe a cough or wheeze without any organic reason, and your skin may feel different, possibly dry. This is an indication that the Lung Qi has possibly been damaged by emotional effects.

When the behaviour of one phase becomes exaggerated, it can deplete or block the other phases. Therefore, if Liver Qi is rebelling, it can deplete the Kidneys, upset the Heart, depress the Spleen and obstruct the Lungs. If you ignore the body signals and fail to rectify the initial problem, it can move on and affect other areas, demanding a longer term of treatment and rehabilitation.

The Five Evils

The body can show effects similar to the climates and cycles of the seasons. Internal conditions correspond to climatic effects, which can be related or unrelated to the external environment.

Chinese medicine is aware of Five Evils that can cause pathology in the body. These Five Evils are Wind, Heat, Damp, Dryness and Cold.

Wind

Wind is movement, unpredictable; it disturbs the location and direction of things. The Wood Phase, spring, is the season of Wind. Wind can find its way into the body, causing unsettling effects on the emotions and disrupting surface and interior circulation of Qi. Wind manifests in the body as jerky movements, dizziness, lack of co-ordination, or symptoms that move through the body, appearing and disappearing without an understandable pattern. External Wind problems are the common cold and flu, with dizziness, aches and pains in joints and muscles, and headache.

Internal problems are vertigo, tremors, headaches, seizures, strokes and emotional instability. Wind can penetrate the defensive Qi and allow other Evils, such as Damp, Dryness and Cold, to enter the body.

Internal Wind is due to a disharmony of the Liver meridian. Extreme heat, due to a high-temperature disease, enters the Blood and generates Wind. Maciocia likens it to the wind generated by a large forest fire.* Liver Yang or rising Liver Qi cause heat and can manifest as internal Wind if allowed to continue without treatment. Deficient Blood creates empty spaces within

* Maciocia, *The Foundations of Chinese Medicine*, p. 296.

the Blood vessels. These empty spaces are taken up by internal Wind.

Heat

Heat accelerates metabolism, dilates blood vessels and activates circulation. Heat rises and moves out toward the surfaces. It is the Fire Phase or summer.

Excessive Heat generates inflammation, rapid pulse and fever. The inflammation will be red, swollen and painful. Hot conditions are thirst, dryness, constipation, difficult urination, agitation. There is a desire for cold foods, with an aversion to warm foods, drinks and climates. Heat moving to the surface causes perspiration and may be due to increased metabolic activity, exercise, feverish diseases or eating warm or spicy foods. When heat invades the surface, skin eruptions, red rashes, welts, sores, ulcers, boils and acne can appear.

Sugar, spicy food, alcohol, some B vitamins, thyroid hormones, adrenaline and amphetamines produce Heat.

Damp

Damp is like a stagnant swamp. Its nature is to sink and accumulate, characterised by an abnormal build-up of fluids or excess secretions. The condition presents as swelling, and a sense of fullness and heaviness. Damp collects and coagulates, causing stagnation and obstruction of circulation. It is of the Earth Phase or late summer. Evidence of Damp shows in a sluggish feeling, apathy and dullness, or on the surface as oily skin, sticky perspiration, subcutaneous oedema (fluid build-up under the skin surface) and swollen joints.

Internal Damp presents as phlegm and abundant discharge of mucus; water retention and oedema of the abdomen and extremities; heaviness of the head and limbs; dull pain and lethargy.

Dairy products, starchy and glutinous foods, steroids, birth-control pills, watery fruits (melons, grapes, etc.) and vegetables (cucumbers etc.) generate Damp.

Damp is usually accompanied by Cold, Heat or Wind. In Damp Cold, the circulation is constricted; there is aversion to the cold, stiffness and soreness of the muscles and joints, and fatigue.

Damp Heat conditions are red, painful swellings, thick purulent discharge, blisters (herpes and shingles), and inflammations (cystitis, jaundice and bronchitis). Any sore or abscess with pus or fluid indicates Damp Heat.

Sugar, alcohol, fatty and fried foods create Damp Heat.

Damp Wind causes swelling that appears and disappears (hives), bubbly phlegm, and itching, oozing sores and ulcers. In extreme cases Damp Wind can obstruct the brain, causing seizures, strokes, lack of co-ordination, vertigo, and muddled thinking.

Dryness
The nature of Dryness is to wither and shrivel, damaging fluids and causing dehydration. Dryness is of the

Metal Phase or autumn. Dryness can be seen in brittle hair and nails, cracked and wrinkled skin and mucous membranes, irritated eyes, dry stool or constipation, lack of perspiration, and scanty urine.

Internal Dryness occurs with body fluid damage caused by Heat, profuse perspiration, prolonged diarrhoea, excessive urination and loss of blood.

Hot spicy foods, stimulants, diuretics and antihistamines result in Dryness.

Cold

The nature of Cold is to slow things down and so depress metabolism and retard circulation. Winter and the Water Phase relate to Cold. A cold attack on the surface of the body causes skin and muscle contraction, shivering and goose bumps. Cold can also occur due to a deficiency of Yang (metabolic heat) or the ingestion of cold foods, drinks or medicines.

Chronic or prolonged illness, poor diet and exposure to a cold climate (such as air conditioning) can lead to a depletion of Yang, causing Yang to be overcome by Yin and Cold to predominate within the body.

Refrigerated, raw foods and chilled drinks are Cold, including ice cream and iced liquids. Medications such as antibiotics, aspirin and Vitamin C have a Cold nature.

The Stomach depends on the digestive fire to break down and process food, and so Cold foods and medicines weaken the digestive system. The resulting effect of Cold on the digestion is weakness of the immune system, causing asthma, colitis, arthritis, eczema and candidiasis.

Cold can lead to stagnation of Blood and Fluids which congeal into lumps or masses of localised pain and tenderness.

Emotions

The emotions are associated with the Five Phases, and in excess they can cause imbalance in the body. The Five Emotions are Anger, Joy, Melancholia, Sorrow and Fear.

Anger

When Anger is predominant, one feels frustration, causing volatile and erratic behaviour and affecting the circulation of Qi and Blood. Problems resulting from this are ulcers, haemorrhoids and migraines.

Joy

Constant stimulation can cause Joy to be dominant, resulting in extremes of emotions from heightened joy (hysteria) to anxiety, insomnia and despair. Conditions that can occur from a manifestation of Heat and overzealous Joy are hypoglycaemia (low blood sugar) and anorexia.

Melancholia

Melancholia or deep contemplation, fixating on worrisome thoughts and ideas, even obsessiveness, can lead to a suppression of Qi, Blood and Fluids. The conditions may appear as lethargy, poor digestion, heaviness and flabbiness.

Sorrow

If sorrow becomes overwhelming, it leads a person to detachment from others and their own feelings, causing vulnerability. Conditions caused include asthma, constipation, and emotional and physical detachment.

Fear

Fear is a protective element of survival but in extremes it results in alienation, the need to be alone, and a belief in the lack of safety in this world. Fear in extreme can dispirit one and cause arthritis, deafness and senility.

The Consultation

We will now look at what to expect at a consultation with a practitioner of Traditional Chinese Medicine.

Initial Consultation

This introduction to TCM will be a lengthy process, as the practitioner must gauge the reasons and causes of the problem on all parts of the body. TCM is holistic and the practitioner is interested not only in the presenting problems but also the effects they are having on the internal, external and emotional aspects of the person.

A detailed history is gathered, looking back at previous illnesses, operations, injuries and traumas, because these may be precursors for the problem at hand. A current history is then taken of how the presenting problem is affecting you and your emotions.

Further information is needed in regard to menstrual cycle—colour and flow of blood, days of bleeding, any clotting or pain, emotions, cravings, tastes in mouth, pre- and post-menstrual effects. The smell, colour and texture of faeces are important, as well as urine output and its smell and colour.

Finally, the practitioner asks to see your tongue (please do not scrub beforehand), and feels your pulse.

Tongue Diagnosis

The tongue is considered one of the most reliable and useful indicators of health in the individual. The tongue is characterised by its colour, texture, moisture, size and shape. A healthy tongue fits the mouth; it is smooth, moist, pink and firm, with a thin white coating covering the upper surface.

The tongue is divided into areas relating and reflecting systems of the body, as shown in Figure 9.

A pale, enlarged tongue with teethmarks on the edges (indicating that the tongue is bloated and pressing on the teeth) and a greasy white coat is associated with Damp. A red tip and dry tongue may indicate that the Heart is not balanced. Sometimes this is an indication of insomnia or difficulty getting off to sleep, with many thoughts going on in the head; this indicates that Shen has flown from its residence in the Heart. Red sides on the tongue show Liver Qi imbalance, which can also affect the Heart and possibly the Spleen.

External factors, such as smoking, coffee and alcohol, affect the tongue and may mask its true state in diagnosis.

The Pulse

Pulse is another vital diagnostic tool in TCM. Its significance is complex, and many years are needed to master all its intricacies.

There are three pulses on each wrist, corresponding to a particular meridian and organ system, as shown in Figure 11. Each pulse point has three levels to it. The left pulse reflects Heart, Liver and Kidney, whereas the right pulse reflects Lung, Spleen and Kidney Yang. As many as thirty-two pulse qualities are described in the classical texts, each indicating a particular type of disturbance. For instance, wiry pulse is a long pulse which feels stiff and tight-stretched like a wire. Hence, if the Liver position for the pulse shows as wiry, Liver Qi is rebellious. Migraine is an example of rebellious Liver Qi.

The Diagnosis

I regard the history-taking and diagnosis of tongue and pulse as a form of detective work, where I find many conflicting or individual symptoms which, put together, give a full picture of the problems and where they are coming from.

Referring to the Five Phases, one can see the movement through the body and systems if one area is imbalanced. I see this as a process similar to peeling an onion: each layer reflects the movement of the condition down to the root of the problem.

Some clients complain of old symptoms recurring years after the original complaint has completely disappeared. Until we get to the core of the problem,

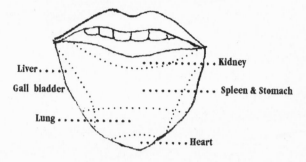

Figure 9. Areas of the tongue and corresponding meridians.

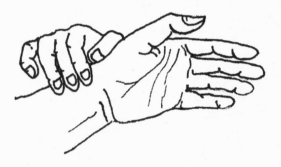

Figure 10. The correct position for taking the pulse.

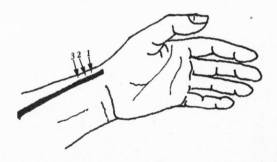

Figure 11. Chinese medicine distinguishes three pulses on each wrist.

there will be movement through all phases to the original problem or condition. Once the core of the condition is treated, further health and well-being can be maintained by lifestyle changes and diet.

This process may seem long: it may only take a few treatments to reach the root, or it may take many, depending on the length of time the client has lived with the problem. I have found that if my clients are prepared to take some responsibility and change even part of their diet, this supports the treatment and speeds things along.

PARTICULAR CONDITIONS

Menstruation

The main meridians functioning at menstruation are Spleen and Liver. Spleen creates blood from food digested in the stomach from Nutritive Qi. Liver stores blood ready for your monthly cycle and other body needs.

A normal cycle is 28 days, and within TCM terms there should be no bloating or emotional highs or lows prior to bleeding. The period should be pain-free, bright red in colour, free-flowing without clots. Bleeding generally lasts for three to five days and should not be accompanied by mood swings or lethargy.

This is the ideal but, because of the demands of our lifestyle and environment, few women experience periods which are pain-free and easy. The main problems encountered in the menstrual cycle are pain, bloating, mood swings, headaches, clots, breast distension and PMT (pre- or post-menstrual tension).

Menstrual disorders are amenorrhea (no bleeding), dysmenorrhea (pain), endometriosis, menorrhagia (excessive bleeding), irregular menstrual cycles, de-layed menstruation and early menstruation. Table 4 on page 42 shows the conditions that are associated with them.

Pain

Painful periods (dysmenorrhea) are usually caused by Cold in the uterus restricting the blood flow. They may be accompanied by pallor, cold limbs, nausea, vomiting, headache or dizziness. During bleeding the body is very open, specifically to allow free flow of blood, but this can also make you susceptible to Cold invasion.

Cold may invade the body, for instance, if you swim in cold water during menstruation. Cold and raw foods and cold drinks may also lead to a Cold condition. During menstruation I recommend that warm, cooked foods be taken, as well as *warm* water or drinks. While your are experiencing pain, you should reduce your intake of coffee; if possible, cut it out completely.

Another reason for pain is stagnant Liver Qi. Stagnation implies non-movement, and where there is non-movement of Qi there is no metabolic heat; thus this non-movement triggers the effects of Cold and therefore pain. Liver Qi is aggravated by emotional frustration and anger, and by sour or cold foods. The pain is worse on pressure and may be accompanied by distension.

Deficiency of Blood and/or Qi is another reason for pain. A poor diet may be the main factor, although a long debilitating illness or heavy periods can also cause this condition.

Excessive sexual activity, excessive exercise, high stress and poor diet are other causes of pain, as they all reduce or block Qi.

To treat pain, the application of heat is the easiest method and has the best effect. A hot-water bottle or heat pack to the lower abdomen, or a warm ginger compress is effective. Essential oil of tarragon (12 drops in ½ cup of vegetable oil) applied to the lower abdomen warms the area and helps circulate Qi, Blood and Fluids. When using any heat treatment, remember to remove it before it becomes cold, to stop further Cold effects.

Ginger and cinnamon tea (see page 82) for breakfast and lunch warms the body, but make sure there are no Heat symptoms such as hot flushes or excessive perspiration. Aspirin may contribute to Cold and so it would be wise to choose a painkiller without it. Vitamin C has a Cold nature, so ceasing its use during pain will be useful.

Bloating and Distension
This is a build-up of Fluids due to Damp, usually triggered by a prolonged diet of raw and cold foods, slowing the digestion and interrupting the dispersement of Fluids. Bloating is usually accompanied by lethargy and lack of motivation, and indicates a disharmony in Spleen Qi and Kidney Qi.

Reducing dairy products and eating cooked and warm foods will help to prevent bloating and distension.

Tonic Soup

To support Spleen, Lung and Kidney and to shift and discharge fluid build-up.

30 g cornsilk	½ cup pearl barley
15 g dry mandarin peel	8 cups vegetable stock
1 slice fresh ginger	1 cup chopped fresh
1 bunch fresh parsley	asparagus
30 g Fu Ling (Poria fungus)	1 cup chopped celery

Place cornsilk, mandarin peel, ginger, parsley and fungus in a muslin bag. Add with asparagus and celery to barley and vegetable stock. Simmer for about 30 minutes. Serve warm.

This soup is useful as a stimulant before meals to enhance digestion of the main meal, or as a snack.

Mood Swings

These can occur before, during and after the time of bleeding and sometimes during ovulation. Anger, aggression, weeping for no apparent reason, depression and melancholia can affect you during any of these times. Table 3 on page 25, showing the Five Phases and associated moods and emotions, can indicate where the disharmony is happening. For instance, weeping, which I regard as one form of expression of fear at this time, may relate to Kidney Qi imbalance. By discerning the area or phase affected and adjusting diet and lifestyle, symptoms may be alleviated. Sometimes an understanding of the issues in your life at the time is enough to enable you to deal with these emotions. A sudden change in relationships may cause grief or fear, as will loss of a job. Anger may be appropriate. Awareness of these emotions, I believe, can help in self-discovery and healing. Knowledge is a healing power in itself.

Clotting

Passing of clots with pain and dark purplish blood indicates stagnation of Liver Qi or Blood. If clots occur without pain in bright red blood they may indicate a predisposition to Liver Qi stagnation. Liver Qi holds the blood and lets it go at the end of approximately 28 days in a normal cycle. Possible causes of clotting are inadequate diet, too much raw or cold food, and stress that exhibits as anger or frustration. The use of tampons can also cause clotting. Tampons do not allow free flow of blood. The tampon acts as a dam, absorbing some of the Blood; any that is not absorbed can flow back to the uterus. The Blood that should have flowed clearly out of the body is held in the uterus where it can coagulate into clots. These clots may be held in the uterus till the next period. I have found that sanitary napkins used at night while sleeping can reduce the number of clots and sometimes the pain. If there are no other indications of Liver Qi imbalance or Blood Stagnation, it may be helpful to use sanitary napkins in the first days of heavier bleeding, or at least during sleep.

I will not go into detailed discussion of all disorders of menstruation and the pathologies for them; Table 4 shows the most common. Following this table is a description of reasons for the pathology and self-treatment.

Table 4
Disorders of menstruation

Condition	Explanation	Possible TCM pathology
Menorrhagia	Excessive menstrual bleeding	Injury to Chong Hot Blood Qi Deficiency
Irregular menstruation	Unpredictable cycle	Liver stagnation Kidney deficiency Spleen deficiency
Delayed menstruation	Cycle longer than 29 days	Cold Qi stasis Blood deficiency Phlegm
Early menstruation	Cycle shorter than 28 days	Qi deficiency Hot Blood
PMT	Pre- or post-menstrual syndrome	Liver Qi stasis Qi stagnation Stagnant Fire affecting Liver and Stomach
Amenorrhea	No bleeding	Cold Qi deficiency Blood deficiency
Endometriosis	Pain caused by endometrial tissue	Qi and Blood stagnation

Hot Blood

Heat causes blood to overspill its vessels. External as well as internal Heat may contribute. Hot spicy foods and over-zealous Yang may cause Heat in the Blood.

A woman I treated had Hot Blood from an excessive use of hot spas and saunas after exercise. She did not slow this down during summer, and this combination led to Heat in the Blood. After modifying her exercise programme and reducing the use of the spa and saunas, her periods regulated themselves, although she did need some treatment for a minor Blood deficiency caused from the large loss of blood.

Alcohol and marijuana can also contribute to Heat in the Blood.

Injury to Chong

The Chong meridian is an extra meridian dealing specifically with the pelvic area. Sex during menstruation, or an abortion, can cause injury to the Chong meridian. I have noticed that many women resume their normal lifestyle almost immediately after an abortion. To avoid shock to this delicate area, it is best to have at least one day of complete rest after the operation and slowly resume exercise regimes. To support possible blood loss, soups with bones, especially chicken soup (see Appendix 2), should be eaten for a few days following this procedure.

Qi Deficiency

Qi can become deficient due to the loss of blood and may present with lethargy, dull thinking and weakened immunity. If there is a deficiency of Qi, there will also be a generalised deficiency of the Kidney and Spleen system and so a lack of Blood and Fluids.

If you cannot consult a TCM practitioner, try to create a temporary reduction of stress factors, such as work. In other words, a holiday and correct eating can help to rectify the deficiency. The body's ability to digest food at this time is very low, so six to eight small meals a day are appropriate. Suitable meals are porridge, soups, vegetables, small amounts of chicken and red meat. I suggest that red meat be incorporated into stews or soups to aid digestion without depleting it, and this also builds Blood.

Kidney Deficiency

Indicators of Kidney deficiency are soreness of the lower back and knees, aching calves, and possibly soreness or aching in the soles of the feet. The Kidney is most susceptible to Cold, and cold food and drinks—especially refrigerated—deplete this system. Frequent births can be depleting, as can sexual exhaustion. A Cold environment may also be a contributing factor to Kidney deficiency. Air conditioning is an external factor that can affect Kidney Qi.

A major Kidney "gate" or point is on the soles of the feet. Wearing socks as much as possible instead of bare feet on cold floors will greatly enhance the Kidney Qi and protect it from Cold.

Stagnant Liver Qi

Excesses of emotions such as irritability, frustration and anger can cause Liver Qi stagnation. Other symptoms may be the sensation of a lump in the throat; distension of flanks, groin or breast regions; lumps in the neck; and clotting during menstruation. Liver Qi may invade the Spleen, causing vomiting, nausea, abdominal distension, flatulence and diarrhoea.

To calm Liver Qi, avoid alcohol, coffee, spicy foods,

food additives and preservatives. This condition is better managed by lifestyle changes than by diet, although certain foods may assist appropriate movement of Liver Qi: basil, bay leaf, beetroot, cabbage, coconut milk, spring onions, and peaches.

The emotions of anger and frustration are sometimes related to stress, whether at work, in relationships or at home. Appropriate management of time and stress should be investigated, along with possible short-term counselling to understand the use of anger. I see Liver Qi as the "great motivator". It helps get things done, and many people thrive on stress to achieve goals. I prefer to harness Liver Qi energy and make it work for me rather than let it rule me. The same can be said for anger: do not try to sedate or restrict its flow, but be aware of what triggers it and use it to your benefit.

Spleen Deficiency

Spleen deficiency can result from Liver Qi stagnation and from dietary imbalance. Its symptoms are poor appetite, abdominal distension, slight epigastric pain relieved by pressure, loose stools, and fatigue. When this occurs, the pure Qi is difficult to extract from digested food and so other areas such as Blood and Fluids are affected. Damp is a condition of Spleen deficiency and is indicated by conditions such as leukorrhea (abnormal vaginal discharge), oedema (fluid build-up), gastritis (inflamed stomach), enteritis (inflamed bowel), nephritis (inflamed kidneys) and colitis (inflamed large bowel).

All foods must be cooked (well-digested) and

warm. Fruits are allowed only if cooked, along with yellow vegetables (pumpkin, carrot, sweet potato) and small amounts of lamb, chicken or pork. No sweets are allowed, nor are fried or greasy foods. Milk and dairy products should be replaced with soy products. If Damp is allowed to continue without treatment, undigested food can lead to Phlegm in the body.

Spleen deficiency can also occur due to long terms of inactivity, affecting sedentary people and those involved in thought rather than action. If these periods of inactivity can be interspersed with physical activity or exercise, it will go a long way in activating Spleen. Our environment is also a contributing factor, with damp in winter and high humidity in summer. Correct diet and exercise are the major protectors of Spleen Qi.

Blood Deficiency
Haemorrhage or prolonged illness may cause Blood deficiency. Symptoms include vertigo, thinness, emaciation, blurred vision, numbness of the extremities, dry skin and hair and pale face. Blood deficiency is usually the result of Spleen and Kidney imbalance due to a weak digestion caused by incorrect and deficient diet or emotional stress.

The diet needs to be regular, incorporating three meals a day, supplemented with blood-building foods such as leafy green vegetables (a good source of iron), liver (pâté), small amounts of red meat, Chinese red dates (*hong zao*), chicken and other soups, baked beans and peanuts. Blood deficiency, if not checked, can lead to infertility.

Qi Stagnation

When Qi is blocked, it is not able to support Blood and Fluids. This condition is brought on by emotional distress, especially grief, worry and depression.

Stagnant Qi responds well to gentle exercise such as Tai Chi or Yoga. Heat to the abdomen is also useful. Relaxation exercises can help, and a particularly useful and calming exercise is described here. It helps to house Shen (the mind) in the Heart and facilitates harmonious circulation of Qi. Try to do this exercise every evening for about 10 minutes.

Calming Exercise

Hold palms of the hands to the abdomen just below the umbilicus (belly button) and with relaxed breathing, relax and allow all thoughts and awareness to go to the area where the palms are resting. Be aware of the rise and fall of the abdomen without concentrating too hard on this area. After a while you may note that the abdomen is rising and falling gently with the breath.

Phlegm

Phlegm is a form of Damp that is thicker and harder to move and sometimes includes undigested food. It occurs when Damp is heated from within, causing it to coagulate and thicken into Phlegm. It usually settles in the Middle Burner or pelvic area, obstructing the flow of Qi, Blood and Fluids. Treatment of Phlegm is similar to treatment of Damp in relation to dietary and lifestyle changes. All foods must be cooked (well-digested) and warm. Fruits are allowed only if cooked, together with sweet and yellow vegetables and meats: pumpkin, carrot, sweet potato, small amounts of lamb, chicken or pork. No sweets are allowed, nor are fried or greasy foods. Milk and dairy products also need to be restricted and replaced with soy products.

Stagnant Fire

This affects Liver and Stomach. It is characterised by irritating pain in the breast during menstruation, a sensation of heat in the breast area, and thirst. Leukorrhea (unusual vaginal discharge) usually accompanies these symptoms.

Eliminate all Heat-forming foods and drinks such as alcohol, spicy foods, red meats, deep-fried foods, sugar, fresh fruit, and avoid tobacco and marijuana. Do not incorporate cold foods and drinks because these will only deplete Spleen Qi further. Invalid foods such as cooked vegetables, barley, white rice, porridge and soy products are appropriate.

Infertility

Infertility in women can be either primary or secondary. Primary infertility is due to a number of factors: intact hymen; abnormality of the vagina, cervix or uterus; blockage of the fallopian tubes; salpingitis; or some abnormality of the ovaries causing hormonal imbalance or anovulatory cycles (nonovulation). Secondary infertility refers to the problem in which a woman has had one successful pregnancy and becomes infertile, sometimes due to uterine infections.

If the menstrual cycle is about 28–30 days, then ovulation occurs between Day 12 and Day 16 after the first day of bleeding.

Infertility in TCM terms looks at the issues from an energetic point of view, with causes such as:

- abnormality of the uterus
- stagnant Blood in Lower Burner
- deficiency or excess in pelvic area
- cold or heat in pelvic area
- imbalance of fluid circulation
- extreme obesity
- emaciation as in anorexia
- weakness
- jealousy.

Most of these conditions relate to menstrual disorders and so it follows that the menstrual problems need to be attended to before any effort is made to achieve conception.

From my experience, the most common reasons for infertility are Cold in the uterus, Blood deficiency, Damp, Phlegm, Qi or Blood stagnation, and decline of Jing (Kidney Qi deficiency) Most problems in infertility need to be addressed by treatment with herbs and/or acupuncture.

The male partner needs to be assessed also to eliminate any problems interfering with his fertility. Areas that may affect his level of fertility are sperm count, motility (movement) and morphology (deformed sperm) and, in TCM terms, Kidney Yang deficiency, impotence from injury to Heart and Spleen, Damp Heat in Lower Burner, and Kidney Yin deficiency.* The male partner should be tested first if there is difficulty in conception. Most areas of male fertility can be corrected simply and the methods of determining the problem are a lot simpler with fewer invasive procedures than are required for women.

There are areas that both partners can work on that will greatly enhance fertility.

Lifestyle
Overwork is a major factor in male and female infertility. It depletes the vital essence, causing mainly tiredness, lethargy, and sometimes decrease in libido and impotence.

In my experience, reducing the stress level (physical and emotional) at work seems to work wonders. For conception to occur, an ovum must be produced and released for a sperm to fertilise. Both sperm and ovum need to be released. I have found that with a high-stress job there is a general inability to let energy go because energy is controlled to allow optimum functioning.

This non-release factor can cause constipation, insomnia and infertility. Substances such as alcohol and drugs (prescription and recreational) help to bring the energy down and also damage the Spleen and Kidney and Liver Qi. Overwork, stress and substance abuse become a vicious cycle slowly depleting the whole body.

*Recently there have been some positive results in regards to the allergic response of sperm to female secretions. The use of TCM herbs has helped achieve pregnancy in this condition: Cathay Herbal Labs, *Newsletter*, Summer 1996.

The body must be relaxed and calm to allow the function of release to occur.

Excessive exercise, as well as excessive sexual activity, causes stress on the Qi. In the male, sperm needs to build up to achieve optimum levels. Sex every day depletes the number of sperm and also injures Kidney Qi. Sex every second day at least allows the sperm-count to build up and allows Kidney Qi to build some reserve. To help conception, I suggest abstinence for at least four days after bleeding stops and then sex every second day for eight days. This covers the most likely time for ovulation, Days 12–16 of the cycle, so there is a good store of sperm for each ejaculation. Sperm can still be active up to 24 hours after ejaculation.

Diet

This is the integral factor for healthy and optimum functioning of the body and all levels of Qi. To support fertility, the Spleen needs help to produce Blood to feed the uterus and to maintain correct functioning of the menstrual cycle. When Spleen Qi is deficient due to a Cold diet, usually Damp becomes prevalent. Damp blocks the channels of the pelvic area, delaying or stopping correct movement of Qi, Blood and Fluids. If food intake is low, it may cause a Blood deficiency. If the body is not well nourished, it will have no ability to support itself, let alone enough for conception and pregnancy. Cold in the uterus and the pelvic area can be caused by Damp or Qi stagnation due to the intake of cold and raw foods and drinks, or climate.

To support conception, food intake must support Spleen and its ability to transform essence to blood and Qi. This food must be warm, cooked and energetically Spleen type (see under Diet, page 106). Kidney Qi also responds favourably to the warm and cooked diet and less so to raw, cold or refrigerated foods and drinks.

At least three good meals should be eaten each day, beginning with a large breakfast and ending with a smallish dinner. Cease or significantly reduce alcohol, coffee, spicy foods, fried and greasy foods, cigarettes and marijuana.

Ovulation
There are numerous tests that determine ovulation. A simple method is to take your oral temperature, before rising from your bed, before having a warm drink, every morning for a number of menstrual cycles. Ovulation causes the temperature to rise slightly by 0.2–0.6 degrees Celsius over a period of five days. Figures 12 and 13 show an example of a temperature chart and how to plot your temperature.

Day 1 of a period is the first day of bleeding, and each day is sequentially numbered till a new cycle of bleeding begins (Figure 12).

Bleeding can be marked with an asterisk on the temperature level of the chart. When bleeding ceases, mark the chart with a dot at the temperature level appropriate to the thermometer reading for that morning. Sex can be indicated by X. The temperature chart for a normal cycle should be like the one shown in Figure 13.

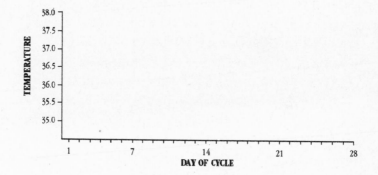

*Figure 12. A chart for recording temperature to
determine the time of ovulation.*

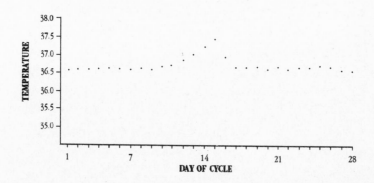

*Figure 13. A typical chart shows a rise in
temperature on ovulation.*

When the temperature rises, around Day 12 to 16, this is a reasonable indication that ovulation is occurring. Ovulation usually occurs through alternate fallopian tubes each month, and sometimes misses a month. This is why it is a good idea to take a chart over a few months to see the pattern of ovulation.

Some women experience a dragging or pulling discomfort on ovulation; others notice some distension. Another indicator is a white mucous discharge which has no unusual smell. If you plan to take this chart to a TCM practitioner, other comments in regard to your emotions, menstrual cycle problems and pain would be useful.

Pregnancy and Birth

Pregnancy is accompanied by a number of physical changes, mainly the cessation of menses (periods), an increase in vaginal excretion, a change in the pigmentation of the external genitalia, enlargement of the breasts, and a darkening of the nipple and surrounding areola.

Although the cessation of menses is a good indicator of possible pregnancy, some women have a slight "show" of blood every month throughout their pregnancy. Usually this is not an indication of problems unless other symptoms, such as pelvic pain, are present.

The pregnancy is divided into three equal sections of three months, known as trimesters.

First Trimester

During this trimester many women experience morning sickness. Despite the name, it may occur in the evening or throughout the day. Morning sickness is usually experienced as nausea, sometimes with vomiting and/or dizziness.

Morning sickness in TCM terms is considered to have three possible causes: Liver Qi rising, giving acid vomiting, regurgitation, belching, a bitter taste in the mouth and sometimes congestion in the chest; Yang Qi rebelling upwards, causing a thirst for water, vomiting, dizziness, tinnitus (ringing in the ears), insomnia, palpitations and chest congestion; or Phlegm Damp obstructing the stomach, with symptoms of acid regurgitation, vomiting of watery substance, dizziness, palpitations, chest congestion, and food seems tasteless.

Simple remedies can sometimes alleviate these symptoms. A cup of weak peppermint or ginger tea with a light snack of, say, toast, before getting out of bed helps many women and alleviates the nausea. Gentle kneading of the abdomen with the palms of the hands can also relieve nausea. Gently sucking *umeboshi* plums and then eating the flesh also seems to help. Morning sickness can be very upsetting and some women become quite anxious with it. Calming and relaxation techniques are useful, and sometimes sitting quietly with the palms of the hands over the abdomen can help to alleviate anxiety. The food and liquid intake must be watched because the vomiting and nausea make eating difficult. There is the possibility that a drain of vital essence will affect the mother later in the pregnancy. Small amounts, often, is the appropriate regime.

Overheating can occur from excessive exercise or from alcohol (its nature being warm to hot) and hot, spicy and fried foods, so the latter should be eliminated from the diet. If the body becomes overheated, it makes it difficult to hold the blood and the foetus. Heat causes Blood to overspill its vessels. Heat depletes the Spleen and stops its normal function of holding up. Too much Heat causes overheating of the Blood and may cause miscarriage.

Second Trimester

The enlargement of the abdomen is noticeable. Usually the morning sickness has subsided, and the mother-to-be appears more content and relaxed. A "quickening" or "fluttering" of the foetus is felt as it begins to move more distinctly. During this trimester it is appropriate to review lifestyle and diet and to make changes, ready for the last trimester. Lifestyle changes could include the reduction of physical and emotional stress (if possible), and classes in Yoga. The diet should incorporate foods to build Blood and Kidney Qi as well as to support Spleen Qi. See under Diet, page 106, for suggestions of such foods.

Third Trimester

This is the time for the foetus to grow stronger and larger, preparing for its birth. During this time the mother-to-be experiences stronger movements and practice contractions. Frequent urination and constipation are typical problems during the third trimester, with the growth of the foetus putting pressure on the bladder and rectum. Posture can have a favourable effect: stand straight, and tuck in your bottom; if it pushes out it will push the abdomen out, putting more weight on the lower back.

This trimester is a time for the baby to gather strength; it should be used by the expectant mother to do the same. Regular gentle exercise, relaxation exercises, correct diet, and plenty of sleep maintain a stable and smooth circulation of Qi. It is also appropriate to avoid lifting heavy objects, and to abstain from alcohol, smoking, and the use of recreational drugs.

Prenatal Exercise

This is an excellent exercise to help stretch the peritoneum area, strengthen the muscles of the abdomen, pelvis and inner thighs, and relax the lower back.

Lie on your back with your knees bent and dropped open to the sides, with the soles of the feet together. Draw your bent legs as close to the body as comfortable, place your arms by your sides. Inhale deeply.

On exhaling, tighten your abdominal muscles to flatten your belly, and feel your spine lengthen and flatten to the floor. Press your heels together and let your knees move toward each other a little. This stretch will be felt in the inner thighs. Inhale. Relax your hips and let your knees drop open.

Repeat six times on a daily basis.

Table 5
Disorders of pregnancy

Condition	Possible TCM Pathology
Abdominal pain	Cold
	Qi deficiency
	Food stagnation
	Wind Cold
	Qi stagnation
Threatened miscarriage	Kidney deficiency
	Liver stagnation
	Spleen deficiency
	Cold
	Heat
Vaginal bleeding	Hot Blood
	Wind Heat
	Spleen or Stomach deficiency
	Blood deficiency
Habitual miscarriage	Qi and Blood deficiency
	Blood Heat
Oedema	Spleen deficiency
	Kidney deficiency
	Qi stagnation
Eclampsia	Hot Blood Wind
	Blood deficiency
	Wind Heat
	Qi deficiency
	Phlegm stagnation
Dysuria	Qi deficiency
	Kidney deficiency
	Damp Heat
	Qi stagnation

Pain

Pain may be felt in the abdomen after conception. It may occur anywhere between the chest and abdomen, within the lower abdomen or in the lower back area. If this pain is intermittent and is not accompanied by bleeding, fever or any other unusual symptom, then it may be the stretching of ligaments and muscles that support the uterus. Lying still with feet elevated usually alleviates the pain.

If the pain feels cold and is accompanied by chills, oedema and loose stools, it is called Empty Cold in TCM terms. Applying heat to the area with a hot water bottle will help the pain. Adjust the diet if there has been an excessive use of cold or raw foods and drinks. Ginger and cinnamon tea (see page 82) will help warm internally. You should increase the intake of warm and cooked foods. Chicken soup with white rice or noodles is an excellent food to heat and support Spleen Yang (see Appendix 2).

Qi-deficient pain is marked by a bearing-down sensation, lethargy, pallor, shortness of breath and poor appetite. This condition responds well to TCM herbal treatment. But also look at the aggressiveness of any exercise programme you are taking: was there any heavy lifting, or standing for long periods of time? Taking some time out to relax and eat regularly will also help with this condition.

Food stagnation due to Wind Cold consists of fullness and pain in the upper abdomen, and reduced appetite. Food stagnation is characterised by regurgitation, fullness and bloating, and constipation or loose stool with an offensive smell. Wind Cold causes painful joints, headache, and possibly a cough with high fever. These symptoms may also be called flu, and are best treated with herbs. Additionally, your diet can be adjusted to incorporate barley, white rice, and cooked foods such as pumpkin, carrot and sweet potato. Ginger tea with chopped spring onions will help open and move the Cold. Peppermint tea is also useful.

Threatened miscarriage, vaginal bleeding and habitual miscarriage are problems best treated by a health practitioner. Awareness of what can trigger these conditions and adjustment to lifestyle and diet can prevent them occurring. As Table 5 shows, Heat and certain Qi deficiencies can cause these conditions. See under Diet, page 106, for ways to remedy these deficiencies.

Oedema

Oedema, the build-up of fluids in the tissues of the body, can be caused by Spleen or Kidney deficiency and so diet can be the major instigator of this condition. If Spleen is deficient, it is not able to transport and transform Water Damp. If Kidney is deficient, it is not able to control water; Fluid builds up, inhibiting transportation of Qi and Blood, resulting in Qi stagnation and Damp blockage. The reduction of salt and fat in the diet, as well as removal of raw and cold foods, can help alleviate the symptoms. Gentle exercise such as swimming and walking helps move Damp. Elevate your feet when sitting, and avoid tight clothes which restrict the flow of Qi and Blood. Extreme or prolonged oedema may lead to hypertension, and prompt attention is needed to prevent eclampsia gravidarum.

Eclampsia gravidarum is a protracted state of Blood exhaustion and Yin deficiency, leading to hyperactivity of Yang. Symptoms are fainting, cramping in the extremities, staring eyes and unconsciousness. Eventually the Blood can be become so deficient that it fails to nourish and moisten the tendons and muscles, causing cramping. This condition can only be treated by a health practitioner, and treatment should be sought urgently.

Dysuria

Dysuria (difficulty in urination or blocked urination) is associated with distension and acute pain in the abdomen. This may be due to the size and position of the foetus putting pressure on the bladder. Posture sometimes alleviates this condition: practise the pelvic rock to ease the pressure.

Pelvic Rock Exercise

Standing flat against a wall, with shoulders straight and pressed against the wall, feel for the small of the lower back. If this is a large gap, indicating the abdomen is pushed out, try to relax the lower back into the wall to reduce the gap.

Do not use diuretics, because they aggravate Damp. Also do not restrict fluid intake, because this may damage the Kidneys. Try to cease cups of tea and coffee (as these act as diuretics). Drink warm water, but do not exceed 2 litres in a day as this will build up Damp. Once more, Spleen and Kidney are affected, and diet may be an indication for this condition. Assess your diet and adjust accordingly, following the suggestions under Diet, page 106.

Labour

Delivery is usually expected 280 days after conception. It is indicated by paroxysmal (wave-like) contractions of the abdomen, and usually a bearing-down sensation in the lower abdomen. As the uterus contracts more, there are stronger bearing-down sensations in the lumbar and abdominal regions, with shorter intervals between each contraction.

There are many strategies to make the labouring woman more comfortable. Heat packs on the lumbar region help to alleviate cramping pains. Warm drinks help to replenish body fluids, and raspberry leaf tea aids contractions. Sucking ice may add to the pain of contractions. Ice or cold drinks slow Blood and Fluids down and so can depress or retard circulation, especially in the pelvic region, and reduce the strength of Kidney Yang. Gravity can help alleviate pressure on the bowel and bladder if the woman kneels on all fours during contractions. The use of certain essential oils has been found beneficial. Lavender is clearly a useful one for calming and soothing. Clary sage, a plant source of oestrogen, is useful in supporting contractions.

A number of points or "gates" on the legs can

facilitate labour. If your birth partner presses on these points with the thumbs, or even holds them firmly, Qi is activated to draw down and release. Your partner must use firm pressure without causing pain, and it would be best for them to practise on themselves beforehand. The points are called Spleen 9 and Spleen 6 (Figure 14), Stomach 36 (Figure 15), Bladder 67 (Figure 16), and Large Intestine 4 (Figure 17).

During labour you may find it difficult to lie still in a position to allow all these points to be used. The best one is Bladder 67, which also helps with pain during contractions. A heat pad applied to Bladder 67 may also help with a difficult labour.

Body fluids may become empty as a result of over-exertion and profuse haemorrhage during delivery, causing a loss of Yin. A few days after delivery, a light fever, aversion to cold and profuse perspiration can occur, but these usually subside after a few days. If you experience these, be aware that it is a time when Cold could enter. Try to protect yourself by changing out of wet clothes as soon as possible, do not sit directly under a fan or air conditioner, and drink warm liquids rather than cold drinks.

Possible disorders during pregnancy are abdominal pain, threatened miscarriage, vaginal bleeding, miscarriage, oedema, eclampsia, and dysuria (inability to urinate). Table 5 indicates possible TCM pathologies for these conditions. Many of them should be treated by a health practitioner, but some suggestions follow to help treatment or to reduce the likelihood of the problem.

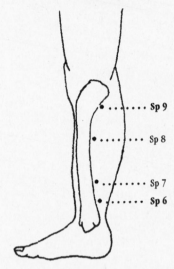

Figure 14. Location of pressure points Spleen 9 and Spleen 6.

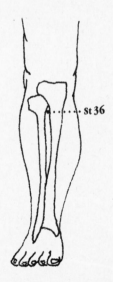

Figure 15. Location of pressure point Stomach 36.

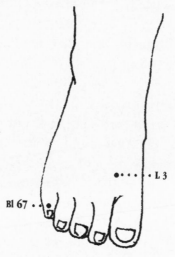

Figure 16. Location of pressure point Bladder 67 and Liver 3.

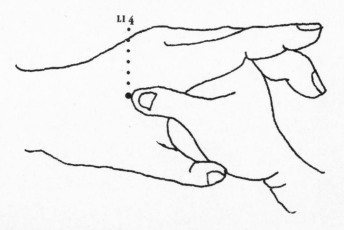

Figure 17. Location of pressure point Large Intestine 4.

After the Birth

Postpartum or after-birth problems are usually due to deficiency. This is the result of Blood or Fluid loss, and it leads to Qi and Blood exhaustion, causing Empty Cold complicated by invasion of Wind.

These conditions can cause pain that responds well to gentle pressure with a heat pack. Warming soups and foods help build Blood and Qi. Rest and warmth are the most appropriate course of action, although it may be necessary for some herbal intervention as well. Constipation may also be a problem. Drink a glass of warm water with a tablespoon of honey in it, at least once a day, to help lubricate the bowel, restoring normal bowel movement.

Breast Feeding

If there is insufficient milk (scanty lactation) it may be due to emptiness of Qi and Blood. A porridge of red beans can be very effective; other Blood-building foods are pea and ham or chicken soup (see Appendix 2). Scanty lactation also responds well to a herbal concoction. Sometimes stress and anxiety resulting from a long and arduous labour may be reasons for the lack of milk. The milk needs to be released or let go to fill the ducts and breasts. Anxiety can slow this natural process of release and restrict the milk flow. Take plenty of rest and do calming exercises, such as the one described on page 47, to help the Qi to move down and release the milk.

Menopause

Menopause is the ending of periods or menses, a naturally occurring part of a woman's life. For many women, it can be the beginning of a new life without the fear of getting pregnant. It often occurs when children are leaving home, so the woman has more time for herself.

TCM looks at a woman's life in seven-year periods. At fourteen years of age, on average, a girl reaches puberty and begins menstruating. At forty-nine years of age (seven times seven) it is said that the Kidney Qi declines, therefore the Chong (pelvic area) is no longer nourished and menstruation ceases. Menstruation is the outward manifestation of Jing and its relationship with Kidney Qi, so with this natural decline of Kidney Qi, menstruation ceases. As the Kidney Qi declines, Spleen Qi also slows down because it is no longer required to produce as much blood. As the Spleen Qi slows down, it affects the digestion: many women find that they gain extra weight, even though their diet and exercise pattern have not changed. In terms of Western medicine, it is good to carry a little extra weight (about 5 kg) during and after menopause as these fatty deposits store oestrogen. Oestrogen declines with menopause, so storing some in fatty tissue helps with some of the unpleasant aspects of menopause such as hot flushes and drying of skin, hair and vaginal secretions.

Most of us know only too well the expected symptoms of menopause due to the extensive media coverage over the last few years. The main issue on which the media focuses is the loss of youth and the ability to conceive. I do not agree that this is a problem. We cannot slow down the ageing process and stay teenagers all our lives: this would be an *unnatural* process. If we have purpose in our lives to make it worth living, menopause is a wonderful experience for most women.

In some societies older, menses-free women are revered for their knowledge, and they shift into a different status within their community during this transition. These women are sought out for their wisdom, but they are also freer than their younger sisters as they no longer have to hold the reins of motherhood. Many women fear a decline of sexual activity after the menopause, but recent research into ageing has shown that this is not true. Sexual activity is an integral part of our lives to death. It may be a little less frequent or slower, but it still happens. I am reminded at this point of a woman in her seventies, whose husband had died about ten years before, who met a man in his sixties. She was amazed that after ten years of inactivity she still functioned as a sexual being. In her terms, she was amazed at the "free flow of sexual juices", as if she were a young woman again.

Our lifestyle to this point may well have an impact on what we experience during menopause. Women who take recreational drugs, drink to excess, smoke, eat incorrectly or poorly, and don't exercise are likely to have a more difficult menopause than more health-conscious women.

Betty Friedan reports in her book *The Fountain of*

*Age** that women who led full and happy lives without a high level of stress did not experience many menopausal symptoms and did not realise they were menopausal until their periods stopped altogether.

If, during your periods, you are diagnosed as having Liver Qi stagnation and no treatment or dietary changes are implemented, this condition may continue with menopause. Conditions during menstruation, if not corrected, will cause difficulties with menopause.

The Liver has a strong relationship to the uterus and the menstrual cycle. Any Liver disharmony will have a strong impact upon menopause. Liver Qi can be affected by anger and frustration, usually caused by stress; whether it be physical stress (work) or emotional stress. Long-term stress can stagnate the Liver Qi and, if not corrected, can lead to pathogenic Heat. Heat occurs if Qi stagnates in one place long enough: it can become hot and ultimately stagnant Fire. Qi can be seen as a source of warmth and energy. If its passage is blocked, Qi continues to move and push against the blockage: this continuous movement of going nowhere builds up Heat. The Heat has nowhere to go naturally, and needs to "vent" or escape. Excessive Heat dries out the Blood and Fluids; this allows Yang to rise to the surface, causing hot flushes, night sweats, headaches, irritability, dry eyes, vertigo and insomnia.

Blood that becomes overheated can spill over and out of its vessels, causing erratic and heavy bleeding

* Betty Friedan, (1993) *The Foundation of Age*, p.140.

during or between periods. This can lead to Blood deficiency. At the time of menopause, less Blood is being produced due to the decline of Kidney and Spleen Qi, and so other organs and areas are affected by the Blood deficiency.

Stagnant Liver Qi can become depressed Liver Fire. This causes painful breasts, a stuffy oppressed sensation in the chest, bitter taste in the mouth, irritability with bouts of depression, and sometimes bleeding gums and toothaches if Fire vents up.

Stagnant Qi can also aggravate the menopause if there is a Spleen or Kidney Yang deficiency. If the Spleen is weak and then invaded by Liver Fire, there may be more Damp and Phlegm, causing oedema, loose stools, obesity, and possibly lumps and growths in the flesh and organs.

Liver Qi stagnation can also affect the Heart. Heart houses the Shen (mind); if Liver and Heart blood become exhausted, Shen will "fly" or be unable to rest. Symptoms are palpitations, insomnia, restlessness, anxiety, poor memory, emotional liability and dreams that disturb sleep.

Conditions common to the menopause are hot flushes, sore eyes, night sweats, insomnia, irritability and depression, anxiety, fatigue, aches and pains, dryness of skin and hair, irregular bowel movements, loss of sense of well-being. We will look at some of these in more detail.

Hot Flushes
These are due to Kidney Yin deficiency and rising

Liver Yang. Hot flushes are usually experienced as a rising of Heat, particularly through the chest and head. Yin is required to control and hold down Yang in the body. If Kidney Yin is deficient, Yang is not being held down and so rises unrestrained to the top part of the body. A sweat or profuse perspiration usually accompanies this rise of Yang. This sweat can exhaust Heart Blood and leads to anxiety, mental instability and palpitations.

Dry or Sore Eyes
These are also caused by rising Liver Yang depleting the Fluids, and the Liver meridian reflects in the eyes.

Night Sweats
Protective Qi controls perspiration and moves quickly and aggressively. At night Protective Qi withdraws to the centre of the body; during the day, it surfaces. Rising body heat forces fluids out to the surface, as in exercise. Night sweats are abnormal, because the body is at rest and not exerting itself. Night sweats indicate Yin-deficient Heat or Fire. Yin is therefore weak and not controlling the night-time or holding down Yang.

Insomnia
Hot flushes and night sweats can cause waking and make further sleep difficult. Usually it is Heat in the Heart causing Shen to fly that causes insomnia. Once more Yang is moving up due to a Yin deficiency. Because the periods have stopped and the body is no

longer creating extra Blood, insomnia may also be caused by Blood deficiency. Blood is Yin and so once more we have a Yin deficiency.

Irritability and Depression

These are due largely to stagnant Liver Qi. Anger and frustration block Liver Qi. This blockage stops Heat flowing correctly, and without correct flow, depression can occur. If the Heat suddenly moves, it will show as fits of anger and irritability. These two problems can occur alternately due to the obstruction of Liver Qi.

Nervousness and Anxiety

Like insomnia, these are related to the Heart. Heat can move Shen from its residence (in the Heart) causing it to fly and flutter away. This can be indicated by many thoughts going on in the head when you are trying to sleep. Blood deficiency linked to Heart can also cause Shen to fly. Palpitations are another sign of Heart Blood deficiency.

Fatigue

Fatigue relates to Qi deficiency and this can be caused by Liver attacking Spleen. Spleen, when deficient, cannot make Blood and Qi, thereby causing a Heart deficiency due to lack of Blood. Qi becomes deficient from the inability of Kidney to grasp Qi and help it flow through the body. Spleen Qi is declining when we are in our forties and so it is necessary to support it as much as possible. Diet and lifestyle changes can help in this support of Spleen.

Qi deficiency has symptoms such as fatigue, listlessness, fluctuations in appetite, mild diarrhoea. If left unchecked, further problems can occur, such as anaemia, dysfunctional uterine bleeding, prolapse of stomach, uterus, bowel or bladder, a tendency to bruising, nausea, and possible gastro-enteritis. These symptoms also show that the deficiency is related to Spleen. If Kidney becomes deficient, symptoms occur such as low backache, sciatica, lack of will-power, loss of sex drive, and frequent urination or urinary incontinence.

Vaginal Dryness
This is due to a Kidney Liver Yin deficiency where body fluids are not directed to the lower body. If Liver Qi is stagnant, the genitals become dry due to Heat in the Liver channel, causing not only dryness but also chronic inflammation and itching.

Osteoporosis
Kidney rules the bones, teeth, head hair, ears and marrow of the spinal cord and brain. Some recent research into TCM herbal formulas shows that osteoporosis can be controlled. The herbs are a classic Kidney tonic formula.*

Treatment for the Problems of Menopause
If you are in an ideal situation, you will have a good diet, moderate exercise and limited stress factors.

---

* Cathay Herbal Labs, *Newsletter*, Summer 1996

Sadly, all these factors are not practised by the average mid-life woman.

Exercise stimulates the Spleen and strengthens the Lungs. Spleen function improves with exercise, helping to move Damp and Phlegm and therefore boost the energy and Qi levels. Lungs when healthy can keep Liver in check, preventing it from rising out of control and affecting other organs. Moderate exercise like walking, swimming or dancing increases bone density in post-menopausal women and helps prevent bone demineralisation or osteoporosis. Yoga and Tai Chi both require stretching which helps to maintain flexibility, keeping muscles and tendons from becoming stiff.

Lifestyle changes, such as ceasing the use of recreational drugs, reducing alcohol consumption and practising stress management, will help ease the adverse affects of menopause. Recreational drugs deplete Kidney Yin and Yang; as this is in natural decline during menopause, these drugs only speed up the process. Alcohol creates Heat and upsets Liver Qi, causing it to flare up.

A regular massage is therapeutic, but if Damp is prevalent an oil-free technique is appropriate because oil can block the surface, locking Damp in. Oil-free techniques such as Shiatsu, Tuina (Chinese massage) or Thai massage facilitate the movement of Damp.

Diet is important in preventing problems of menopause. Foods which support Spleen and Stomach include cooked and warm foods, grains and vegetables, with small amounts of red meat. Cautious use of warming herbs, such as ginger, nutmeg and cinnamon, can aid digestion. It is best to replace milk products with soya products because milk can aggravate Damp. To keep Liver calm, it is suggested you reduce or avoid coffee (both caffeinated and decaffeinated), alcohol, greasy, fried or oily foods, spicy foods (chilli and curries), excessive amounts of red meat and preservatives.

Some foods and herbs contain precursors to oestrogen. The liver (in the Western sense) can change these to oestrogen, helping to keep these levels up during and after menopause. Oestrogen plants include: alfalfa, aniseed, dill, licorice, parsley, red clover, sage, soya beans. Foods which have a high calcium level are: sesame seeds, kelp, cheese, carob, soya beans, parsley, almond kernels, figs, hazelnuts, watercress, dandelion greens, chick peas, broccoli, leafy green vegetables, and lentils. Be careful not to overdo the oily nuts; remember, everything in moderation.

Two herbs that are specifically useful in opening and soothing the eyes are chrysanthemum flowers and wolfberry (*gou qi zi*). Taken as a tea, they help alleviate sore dry eyes. Wolfberry can be eaten in small amounts, which helps in temporary reduction of tiredness.

Essential oils have some excellent effects on conditions of menopause. Oils can be used in a bath, or mixed with aloe vera gel for massage.

For Hot Flushes

10 drops Clary sage
  essential oil
11 drops Geranium
  essential oil

7 drops lemon
  essential oil
2 drops sage
  essential oil

Mix in 30 ml vegetable oil or aloe vera gel, and apply externally.

For Day and Night Sweats

4 drops grapefruit
  essential oil
4 drops lime
  essential oil

or 4 drops sage
  essential oil
4 drops thyme
  essential oil

Use either combination daily in a warm bath.

For Water Retention and Bloating

2 drops fennel
  essential oil
2 drops juniper
  essential oil

or 6 drops lemon
  essential oil
2 drops peppermint
  essential oil

Use either combination daily in a warm bath.

Migraine

Migraines seem to affect women more than men. In TCM terms, this has a lot to do with rising or stagnant Liver Qi. Because Liver has a special relationship with Blood and the menstrual cycle, it can be seen why migraines affect women more often.

Many women experience migraines either pre-menstrually or during their periods, and sometimes at ovulation.

Migraines can affect the head in different areas. Most commonly they affect the sides of the head and behind the eyes. The pain sometimes starts as a feeling of pressure all over the head, and proceeds to throbbing, sometimes described as pulsating or bursting. The headache can be accompanied by nausea, vomiting, irritability, sensitivity to light and noise, and visual disturbances such as light flashes or blurred vision.

Excessive workloads and tension, high consumption of alcohol and coffee, and poor diet contribute to this condition. The headache often occurs on days off, that is, at the weekend. When the tension levels are reduced, this inactivity allows Liver Yang to rise, causing the headache. Alcohol regularly used to help relax after a tense day aggravates Damp and Heat in the Liver channel, causing Heat to rise. Coffee restricts the flow of Blood, Qi and Fluids by constricting the channels. The headache is sometimes caused by this fluid deficiency. The skin over the skull can sometimes feel bloated or spongy: this is due to fluid retention or Phlegm in the tissue of the skull.

If the migraine is experienced during the menstrual period, there will be signs of stagnation such as clotting, dark purplish blood flow, or brown spotting, distension and pain.

Sometimes a simple change of diet helps to alleviate symptoms. A client complained of migraine and other symptoms indicating Cold and deficiency. On further questioning about her diet I found she preferred iced water with ice cubes added. By eliminating the cold and raw elements of her diet and incorporating warm fluids, her migraines were reduced by 50 per cent. Further treatment with herbs reduced the migraines to nil.

Although migraine sufferers need to have treatment to stop the problem, there are number of points that can be stimulated that can help reduce the pain during the attack. Liver 3 and Large Intestine 4 (see Figures 16 and 17 on page 65) are the most common and easily found. If these points are held with the thumb under strong pressure, some of the symptoms of the migraine subside. If pressure over the head is felt, gentle tapping with the fingertips all over the head helps disperse some of the Phlegm or Damp. Rubbing Po Sum oil or Tiger Balm into the temples reduces the pain temporarily. Cut out coffee and alcohol completely.

I have noticed that excessive amounts of fruit juice can also trigger a migraine. Fruit juices are high in sugar, which is heating, affecting the Liver Yang and allowing it to rise. One glass of orange juice is equal to about three oranges, so one or more glasses of cold

orange juice per day is an overdose of sugar and encourages Heat to rise. It is best to cut out fruit juices
completely for at least a month. If you feel you need
fruit juice, slowly introduce it back into your diet, but
dilute it by half with water. Try not to exceed three
glasses a week. Chocolate can sometimes trigger migraine, perhaps because of the Heat it generates, as
well as causing Damp. Sometimes chocolate helps a
migraine; in this case the migraine could possibly be a
deficient form rather than a stagnant form.

Liver is the main area affected by tension, anger
and overwork. It is also the main reason for migraines.
Diet and lifestyle changes can help restore Liver Qi
dramatically.

Herpes

Herpes is a Damp Heat condition affecting the Liver
channel. Herpes, more commonly known as cold sores,
appears as blister-like sores around the lips. In genital
herpes, similar blister-like sores affect the genital area.

Herpes is a viral infection, and once in the body
it cannot leave. It may be dormant for long periods,
giving the impression that you are no longer infected.
Anyone with herpes is aware that stress can trigger an
outburst. This is an indication, in TCM terms, that the
Liver channel is affected. The Heat from Liver stagnation causes the Fluids to congeal into Phlegm. Phlegm
and Damp accumulate, restricting the normal flow of
Qi and Blood and causing the oozing of Phlegm. At its
worst, it can cause ulcerations. These open sores
allow invasion of Wind, Cold or Heat. Protective Qi is

unable to heal the sores normally. This is the cyclic nature that some sufferers report with herpes.

Herpes can be kept under control by appropriate diet: heat-causing elements are reduced, and cold and raw foods are kept to a minimum. The cold and raw foods create Damp, and hot, spicy, greasy foods heat the Damp to congeal into Phlegm. Stress needs to be minimised because it depletes the immune system. Cut out alcohol completely. Reduce dairy products and incorporate more soya products in the diet. Chocolate also seems to be a strong trigger, possibly because of the dairy ingredients, but chocolate itself is also warming.

During an outbreak, cleanliness is a high priority. A combination of essential oils of bergamot and lavender applied directly to the sores can be beneficial. Bergamot is an excellent skin antiseptic and deodoriser and a calmative: it keeps the area clean and also relieves the hot burning itch. Lavender is antiviral and analgesic, and it has a cooling effect.

For Herpes

6 drops bergamot
essential oil

6 drops lavender
essential oil

For genital herpes, use daily in a warm bath, or combine with ½ cup aloe vera gel and apply to the genital area every 4 hours to reduce pain.

For cold sores, apply (undiluted) to the sore with a cotton bud.

A herpes outbreak as cold sores or on the genitals is distressing, and it can be difficult to feel calm and relaxed during this time. Calming music tapes, relaxing baths and gentle Yoga or Tai Chi exercise will help to calm Liver Qi, thereby reducing the length and frequency of recurrent outbreaks. Chinese herbs appear to have an excellent effect and can help move Damp and calm the Liver. These herbal formulas should not be taken continuously: it is best to seek out a TCM practitioner in regard to dosage and duration of use of these herbs.

Common Cold

The common cold is an invasion of either Cold Wind or Wind Heat. It is characterised by headaches, nasal obstruction, sneezing, nasal discharge, aversion to cold, alternating fever and chills or fever alone, and sore throat.

Sometimes the first indications are a scratchy throat and sneezing, without any other symptoms.

I have found that catching the cold at this point can stop it from further entering the body; usually the symptoms can be relieved in a few days. At this time, even though you may not feel ill, it is best to stay indoors, rest well, and keep warm. If these symptoms are left more than two days, the cold becomes established and will usually last five to seven days, with or without medication.

By taking a combination of ginger and cinnamon tea three times a day on the first day you can relieve the symptoms and usually stop any further problems. The tea can cause a strong night sweat and when this occurs you should stop the tea. The following day try to keep warm, stay out of drafts, and rest as much as possible.

It is better to take a day off at this point than to take a week off later when the cold has established itself deep in the body.

Ginger and Cinnamon Tea

1 slice fresh ginger or 1   3 cups of boiling water
   teaspoon dried ginger
1 large cinnamon stick
   or 1 teaspoon
   cinnamon

Soak ginger and cinnamon in boiling water.
   Take 1 cup of warm tea three times in the first day of cold.
   Do not continue this for more than 2 days. If a sweat occurs, stop immediately.

Cold can enter the body or invade the Protective Qi defences if you wear wet clothes, especially after exercise or swimming. During winter, which is a time of Yin, protect the vulnerable points of the body, the neck and lower back, from cold. Wear warm clothes, especially around those vulnerable areas. If you are in a heated environment wearing light clothing, when leaving the heat make sure you keep warm with adequate clothing. Even if you still feel warm, the neck and lower back are very open and vulnerable to invasion. Wet hair and open car windows are other ways in which Cold can enter the body.

If the body's Qi is weak from overwork, illness, excessive sexual activity, poor diet or emotional stress, it is far more susceptible to an invasion.

Wind Heat enters through the nose and mouth, usually as a pathogenic agent or virus, and presents as fever, headache and sweating, all Heat manifestations. Chrysanthemum tea and peppermint tea are both useful in cooling and dispersing Heat.

Eucalyptus essential oil is cooling and dispersing, and it moves Phlegm. Used as an inhalant or body rub to the chest and back, it may help to dispel some of the symptoms.

Two useful formulas in pill form help relieve symptoms fairly quickly:

- *Yin Chiao* (without sugar): for flu-like symptoms of Phlegm, Heat and aching joints.
- *Gan Mao Ling*: for the common cold of itchy throat and runny nose.

Another useful remedy is Watermelon Frost for sore throat, toothache or mouth ulcers. Just dab it on the sore area.

Depression

There are numerous clinical forms of depression, but for the purposes of this book I will look at it in general terms.

Depression is generally characterised by extreme sadness, lethargy, insomnia, a lack of will, withdrawal from the activities of life, loss of appetite, and a reduction in the sex drive. Certain conditions in our life cause many of us to experience depression. Sometimes it is due to the lack of control in our lives, or even, in the extreme, to changes of weather. Clinical depression is a state that needs full support by an experienced counsellor or psychotherapist. Traditional Chinese herbs, acupuncture and Shiatsu can help support the psychotherapy.

Depression can be due to a number of factors in TCM: Kidney Yang deficiency, Spleen Qi deficiency, Phlegm, Heart Qi deficiency or Liver Qi stagnation.

Kidney Yang or Yin Deficiency

Kidney Yang is associated with will and drive. Kidney Fire (Yang) is the energy that drives the body and is the force behind the will to live. Fear, shock and guilt may injure the Kidneys, and chronic disease, overwork, excessive physical work and lifting and excessive sexual activity also deplete the Kidney Yang. This condition is characterised by mental and physical exhaustion, depression, lack of will-power and initiative, and a feeling of hopelessness. Everything is too much effort. Kidney Yin or essence deficiency is also caused by these factors and, in women, by too many births or heavy periods over many years.

Kidney Yin deficiency is characterised by feeling mentally and physically exhausted and depressed, with a lack of will-power and initiative. There may also be a lack of desire for sex, or impotence. Kidney-deficient depression can also occur due to the ageing process: as Kidney Qi declines it can cause a deficiency.

Spleen and Heart Qi Deficiency

Worry or pensiveness (deep internalisation) over a long period can injure Spleen and Blood, causing deficiency in Spleen Qi and Heart Blood. This weakens Shen (the mind) and moves Shen from its residence, the Heart. Qi and Blood deficiency is characterised by tiredness, lethargy, depression, insomnia. Because the mind controls thinking and memory, there is poor memory, lack of concentration and slow thinking. Spleen and Blood deficiency can also result in obsessive thinking or phobias because the Spleen controls thinking, intelligence and concentration.

The Spleen Qi deficiency leads to the formation of Phlegm, which mists the mind, causing dull, confused thinking and obsessive thoughts. The Blood deficiency causes insomnia and poor memory, and the person is timid and easily startled.

Phlegm

Phlegm can obstruct or "mist" the mind. This obstruction causes mental confusion, impairing the mind's functions of thought, memory, conceptualisation and understanding. It can be likened to moving through a fog, not knowing where anything is, bumping into things, making you feel lost and unable to orientate yourself. The effects of Phlegm are therefore poor memory, dizziness, poor concentration, slow thinking. There may also be a feeling of numbness and an inability to express emotions.

Stagnant Liver Qi

Stagnant Liver Qi can cause the mind (Shen) to be obstructed, causing moodiness, mental depression, pre-menstrual tension, irritability, frustration, arrogance and impatience. Features of this condition are, initially, confusion due to the stagnation, and secondly, a strong resistance to any change, mental or physical. There are physical symptoms of distension, sighing, belching, tiredness, chest tightness or oppression, irregular periods, clumsiness or breast distension. This condition can be caused by shock or prolonged worry which stagnates Qi. Loss of blood during childbirth, or declining blood or Yin in menopause, can also stagnate Liver Qi.

Preventing Depression

One should live a quiet life with few desires so that one can preserve one's Qi and guard one's mind in order to avoid disease. Thus if emotions are absent and craving is curbed, the Heart is peaceful and there is no fear.*

The recommendations of this Taoist quote are difficult for most of us to attain, but calm thoughts, relaxation and fun go a long way in maintaining mental health.

Two ancient "Formulas for the Mind" are written in the form of a herbal prescriptions, to calm the mind.

---

* Maciocia, (1987) *The Practice of Chinese Medicine*, p. 3.

Xiang Sui Wan

Pill to the likeness of Marrow (Blood).

- *Not thinking too much*: nourishes the Heart.
- *Restraining anger*: nourishes the Liver.
- *Restraining sexual desire*: nourishes the Kidneys.
- *Careful talking*: nourishes the Lungs.
- *Regulating diet*: nourishes the Spleen.

Zhen Ren Yang Zang Cao

The Sage's Paste to Nourish the Internal Organs.

- *Remain indifferent whether granted favours or subjected to humiliation*: makes Liver balanced.
- *Be indifferent whether moving or still*: calms Heart fire.
- *Regulate diet*: does not overburden the Spleen.
- *Regulate breathing and moderate talking*: makes Lungs healthy.
- *Calm the mind and prevent distracting thoughts*: replenishes the Kidneys.

By following these prescriptions and incorporating either Yoga, Tai Chi or Qi Gong into our lives, we can nourish the Heart and calm the Liver. Eat less raw, cold food and more warm, cooked food to support the Spleen and Kidneys. Breathing exercises nourish the Lungs.

To support the process of healing depression, diet plays a strong part. Eat foods to strengthen spleen (see under Diet, page 106), and slowly incorporate gentle exercise into your lifestyle.

Short-term depression can be seen as a self-help

mechanism during a time of pressure or failure. It puts the mind on standby, providing a little time of non-thinking and non-action to allow the mind and body to gain strength to tackle the problems. If your body demands sleep and rest, satisfy that need as a healing action.

This sort of depression can occur during holidays or time off from an extremely busy work life. Finally the body and mind have a moment to relax. Try not to fight it and to listen to your body's needs at this time. Incorporate into your life as much as you can of the "Formulas for the Mind" during this time.

Winter is the time of Yin and therefore minimal action. During winter we prefer to be indoors by a fire, and reduce the amount of exercise. Winter is a time for healing and preparation for the spring and summer months. After prolonged deprivation of sunlight (Yang) we can become more Yin (slower), and in some individuals depression can set in. Long-term sitting and reading, or lack of exercise can deplete the Spleen. As we have already seen with Spleen Qi deficiency, gentle exercise can be useful and helps Spleen keep motivated and moving. Raw and cold foods further deplete Spleen and Kidney, so soups, traditional winter fare, are most appropriate.

When spring arrives with its wind and changeable weather, some find they are easily depressed by the colder days and the wind. Spring is Liver time and the changeability of the weather can easily move Shen from its residence (the Heart). Anxiety, depression and lethargy can be experienced. Although not a great deal can be done about this, understanding why we have these moments makes it easier to cope. People who are prone to Liver conditions and those who have a highly stressed, hyperactive lifestyle seem to suffer the most. Protect Spleen by diet, calm the Liver with Yoga, Tai Chi or Qi Gong and support Lung with meditation and breathing exercises.

Obesity

Excess fat or adipose tissue is viewed as obesity. Fat is Yin, as it is an accumulation of substance and therefore mainly Phlegm and Damp in TCM terms. The Spleen deals with transformation of food and transportation of pure essence that converts to Qi, Blood and Fluids. In Chinese dietary therapy, the treatment of obesity mainly involves the Spleen function of transformation and transportation of body fluids and its distillation of food.

The metabolism begins to slow around the age of forty, due to the lessening of Kidney Fire. Kidney Fire is the source of Spleen Yang or digestive fire. As the kidneys produce less warmth, the body's metabolism slows down, leading to a gain in weight. This happens even though the diet or level of exercise has not changed.

To aid the Spleen Yang or energy in digesting food, food should be easily digestible to keep the digestive fire strong and efficient. Spleen becomes dampened by greasy, fatty and damp foods, and deficient by too many sweet, cold or raw foods. Overeating is also a danger because it can block the Qi mechanism.

A glass of warm water before a meal warms the digestion and helps the digestion of food.

Regular exercise allows the Qi, Blood and Fluids to circulate in the body. A good flow of Qi allows the Stomach and intestines to move the impure essences (faecal matter and urine) downwards for excretion.

Exercise warms the body and the Spleen and Kidney Fire. Usually after exercise is when we notice the need to use the toilet, indicating the strengthening of Spleen's transformation process.

Perspiration during exercise helps move excess Damp, although excessive sweating damages Kidney, Spleen and Lung. Unnatural methods of promoting fluid loss, either by diuretics or sweat-inducing garments, damage the body, cause extreme deficiency and slow the metabolism.

Some diet programmes require you to drink large doses of cold water before meals as a way of filling up. Cold water in large amounts floods the Spleen with Damp. Large amounts of grapefruit or other juices causes the Spleen to become Damp, sodden and deficient.

Fasting is inappropriate within TCM dietary therapy because the Spleen requires predictability of meals. Regular meals keep Spleen Yang functioning. Changes or reduction of meals reduce this fire and therefore slow down the Spleen's function of transformation. Fasting usually requires quantities of fruit juices or cold water, further damaging and damping down the Spleen Yang (Fire).

Certain Chinese herbs optimise Spleen function,

move Damp and support Stomach function. These can be prescribed by a practitioner who will create a formula based on your personal requirements. Once a balance has been achieved with these herbs, the diet can continue to support Spleen and Stomach functions.

Chinese green tea (unfermented tea) is useful in aiding digestion. It strengthens the Spleen, reduces Damp, and promotes drainage of pathological Damp by urination. Moderate amounts of green tea during meals aid digestion. Barley as a weak soup or tea has similar functions. Barley or white rice in soups is an ideal diet food. Soup is served warm with cooked food, therefore supporting Spleen function without draining its energy. The inclusion of barley or white rice moves excess Damp.

To reduce unwanted weight and fat, a diet should be high in fibre and complex carbohydrates. Food should be mostly cooked, warm, and easy to digest, spiced with herbs that aid digestion. Cardamom and ginger are two herbs that disperse Phlegm and Damp and aid digestion. Too much chilli or curries heats Damp, thickening it to Phlegm. Very small amounts of chilli or curry are useful. Once more, moderate use is better than excess.

Foods that promote Damp, such as milk, greasy foods, alcohol and fruit juices, should be avoided or reduced. Cold and raw foods which are hard to digest should also be used minimally. Gentle exercise is useful before a meal, because the digestive fire is high and able to break foods down efficiently.

Urinary Tract Infection

Urinary tract infection (UTI), also known as cystitis or urethritis, is known as painful urination syndrome in TCM. This condition is characterised by frequency, scanty urine, pain, urgency and difficulty. Heat is the most frequent reason for this condition, but is not always the main reason; Damp and Damp Heat, Qi stagnation, Qi deficiency and Kidney deficiency are other causes.

External Damp is a common cause of urinary disease. It penetrates the channels of the legs, flows upwards, and settles in the bladder and pelvic area. Sitting on damp grass, living in a damp environment, wading in water, and wearing wet clothes such as bathers or track-suit after heavy perspiration can be reasons for invasion of external Damp. Women are particularly prone to invasion of Damp after their period or childbirth.

Excessive consumption of sweets, sugar, dairy and greasy foods leads to the formation of Damp. Adding spicy foods and alcohol generates Damp Heat. Excessive sexual activity weakens the Kidney. Kidney Qi deficiency can cause dribbling of urine (incontinence). Old age and chronic long-term illness may lead to Spleen Qi deficiency, causing dribbling of urine or difficulty in urination. Emotional stress can also be a cause, along with one or more of the above.

Excessive lifting or standing can cause stagnation of Qi in the Lower Burner. Blockage of the Lower Burner restricts the flow of Fluids and eventually can lead to Damp. Damp can then obstruct the urinary tract. After a hysterectomy, many women complain of recurring cystitis. This is caused by stagnation of Qi and Blood after a surgical removal of the uterus. The nearest organ, the bladder, is affected.

Some good results have been achieved from drinking unsweetened cranberry juice.* It is useful to drink during the infection and for a few days after. Prolonged use could cause Damp. The silk from fresh corn is another useful herb and it appears to relieve the symptoms of UTI within 24 hours.

For UTI

1 handful of dried corn-silk   1 cup of boiling water

Combine and let stand for 5 or 10 minutes.
Sip slowly.
Take three or four times a day during an UTI episode to relieve pain and heat.

ACMERC, *Newsletter*, Vol. 1, 2 November 1995.

LIFESTYLE

Lifestyle has a large influence on the balance of the Qi flow within the meridians and health of the body.

The emotions and climate have a strong effect on health in the individual. The climatic effects of Wind, Heat, Cold and Damp (humidity) can invade the body. If Protective Qi is deficient, these effects enter the body and cause imbalance to the meridians and ultimately the body as a whole.

Cold is a common invader. By keeping your environment and yourself protected, you can reduce the possibility of cold invasion. Simple steps can help maintain balance. To restrict Cold entering the Kidney channel, wear socks rather than going barefoot. A major Kidney point is situated on the soles of the feet.

The Kidney meridian can be deeply affected by Cold, and protecting this single point will also protect the Kidney. Another point susceptible to invasion by Wind and Cold is Gall Bladder 20 (Figure 18).

These two points are quite large and are called Wind Gate. Simple things, such as drying your hair rather than letting it dry in the wind, protect the vulnerable point from invasion. Wearing a scarf or a high collar protects it from invasion on windy or cold days.

Driving a car with the window down is another way Wind Cold can invade. If Wind Cold invades, particularly through Gall Bladder 20, symptoms such as headache can occur, as well as common cold symptoms. Fans and air conditioners can be another means by which Wind Cold invades. Try to position yourself out of the direct flow of cold air.

Heat can affect the body more subtly, but sudden change of temperature is a common cause. Going from air-conditioned rooms to the outside heat is a probable cause. I recommend appropriate clothes, which are needed to protect the body inside, be shed before going out to the heat; a cotton cardigan is useful for this. Heat can cause heavy perspiration, and if you over-exert by exercising in the heat it can cause a heavy release of fluids, leading to Dryness. Excessive

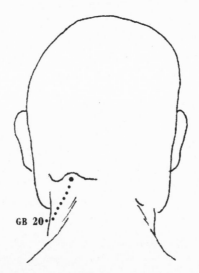

GB 20

Figure 18. Location of pressure point for Gall Bladder 20.

use of saunas and spas can also cause Heat to remain in the body. Heat leading to dryness can affect the Lung, Kidney and Liver channels.

A damp environment can aggravate an already deficient Spleen Qi. A plumber I was treating for a Damp Cold condition complained of arthritic and sciatica-like pain. His work required him to crawl under damp houses to fix plumbing problems. This continuous contact with a cold damp environment caused Cold Damp effects within the body, resulting in the arthritis-like pain. By simply changing his clothes after being in contact with this environment, he reduced the painful condition. A damp house can cause Lung and Damp problems. A combination of efficient heating and ventilation that allows air to circulate freely can usually reduce the problem.

The emotions, in TCM terms, have a strong effect on the meridians. If your refer back to Table 3 on page 25, you will see that particular emotions are associated with particular meridians. This can be used as a guide to understanding these effects.

Liver is affected by anger and frustration. Stress in work or relationships is a major reason for frustration and anger, causing Liver Qi to become excessive. Liver Qi can no longer flow smoothly and, if this condition continues over a long period, the blocked Qi transforms to Heat. If the Heat becomes unblocked and rises, it can affect the person with sudden fits of anger and irritability. Liver Qi rising causes Heat, which has to vent, usually causing headaches—at its worst, migraines. The menstrual cycle is also affected by Liver imbalances; if this is allowed to continue for a long time, it affects Spleen and thereby the digestion.

Spleen is affected by pensiveness or deep contemplation. After long periods of physical inactivity or high intellectual activity, Spleen can become depressed or reduced in activity. Spleen's action is to "hold up", keeping organs in place. A deficient Spleen can exacerbate Damp. Damp affects the flow of Qi, Blood and Fluids. A deficient Spleen slows digestion and the forming of Blood and Qi, and so affects the energy levels. A Spleen-deficient body is affected by lethargy, irregular bowel movement (diarrhoea and constipation), poor digestion, a generalised heaviness of the body, and flabbiness. These effects can be seen in those utilising their intellect above physical needs. Students who study hard without a balance of physical activity find excessive intellectual work can cause Spleen Qi deficiency. Many students neglect to take proper, regular meals and exercise. There is a strong need for those engaged in intellectual pursuits to regulate their diet and exercise to support Spleen function.

Kidney Qi becomes affected through a deficient Spleen's inefficiency in transforming Fluids. Worry depletes Spleen and worry usually feeds fear. Fear depletes Kidney Qi, causing it to descend. When Kidney Qi descends, there are problems with micturition (urinary frequency or incontinence), low backache, tinnitus, and aches along the Bladder meridian of the back, calves and soles of the feet. Fear and chronic anxiety can cause Kidney Yin deficiency, resulting in the rising of Empty Heat within. The Heat gives a feeling of heat in the face, night sweats, palpitations, dry mouth and throat.

Heart is upset by excessive excitement (too much of a good thing) or continuous mental stimulation. Excessive stimulation of Heart can lead to Heart Fire or Heart Empty Heat. Symptoms may be insomnia, dry stool, feeling hot in the afternoon, night sweats, and possibly dreams that disturb sleep.

Sadness weakens the Lungs, but can also affect the Heart by cramping and agitating it so that it pushes towards the Lungs. Because Lung governs Qi, sadness depletes Qi. Symptoms may be breathlessness, tiredness, depression or crying. In women, Lung Qi deficiency can lead to Blood deficiency and amenorrhea.

Exercise is a major help in maintaining health of the meridians and the body. Moderate exercise at least three to four times a week for at least half an hour helps to resolve many problems. Obviously, if you are very Spleen-deficient because of a sedentary lifestyle, gentle exercise such as swimming, walking, Tai Chi or Yoga is appropriate. As the body slowly benefits from this introduction of movement, you can go on to more strenuous forms, such as aerobics, gym circuit or jogging. Jogging is appropriate only on soft surfaces where the impact on joints is minimal. I advise vigorous walking rather than jogging. An exercise regime requires some direction and it is a good idea to seek out a professional in this area to give you directions and to point out what can cause damage.

Acknowledging when you are stressed and what

stresses you is a first step to health. Seek out a reputable stress-management course or counsellor to help pinpoint and manage your stress triggers. It is not possible to eliminate stress, but sometimes an improvement in time management eases it. High expectations can be strong stressors; it is very hard to be the best mother, the best partner, and the best worker all at once. There are areas that can survive for a short while without your full attention. One area may be housekeeping, for instance. Delegate chores to other household members, and feel good about asking for help. Try to ignore a particular area for at least a day. Allow Qi to build up so that you can tackle that area another day.

An emotional time needs to be acknowledged and not pushed aside. If, for instance, sadness or grief is an issue, recognise the emotions. Try to understand why you are feeling these emotions, and take some time to work through them. Make good use of caring and understanding friends and talk it all out. Next time, you can be there for them. It should be obvious that ignoring the emotions can lead to ill health.

Menstruation is a time that can be used to indulge yourself and take time out. During this time do not over-exert yourself with exercise, work or emotions. Be gentle and kind to yourself, and you will feel rejuvenated at the end of the period rather than drained or lethargic. See this time as a gift, not a curse.

Massage is becoming very popular as an aid to reducing stress and calming the mind. If you have a Damp problem, it is best not to have an oil-based massage. The oil blocks the skin and adds to the level of Dampness in the tissues. Oil massage is good for women who find it difficult to relax, who are thin, wiry, hyperactive, always on the go. These symptoms can indicate a type of Wind problem. Oil helps to dampen the effects of Wind, smoothing it out.

The best non-oil massages are traditional Thai massage or Tuina (Chinese massage). Shiatsu is a therapy that incorporates pressure on the points and meridians of the body and is based on TCM. Shiatsu therapists also incorporate diet and lifestyle considerations in the treatment. Shiatsu generally does not use oil in its treatment. Shiatsu is also appropriate for the Wind problem described above. The therapy of Shiatsu is based on the use of meridians and points. It is complementary to herbal and acupuncture treatment. Shiatsu is highly effective on its own, and I find it is useful for those who cannot tolerate acupuncture.

Self-medication

I have deliberately minimised suggestions of a particular herb or formula for a condition. This is because of the effects I have seen in my practice from unwise use of herbs or vitamins. I therefore suggest caution in using supplements.

If you feel you need to take a supplement, do so with thought as to why you need this supplement. Will changes to your diet and lifestyle help alleviate the symptoms? If your diet is inadequate, take the supplement for a month and in that time adjust your diet appropriately. By the time you have finished a month's course, your diet should be beginning to support you and you can stop the supplement.

Any self-medication should be seen as short-term. If the problem still continues after a month, it may be necessary to seek further professional help.

Herbs should be respected for their abilities, strengths and weaknesses. Ideally, the advice of a TCM practitioner advice should be sought before a self-medication regime is started. Long periods of use can change the movement of Qi and injure the body. Chinese medicine uses herbs to bring about change; once that change has occurred, diet and lifestyle changes can support well-being. Moderation is the key to all areas of your life.

Ginseng

This common herb can be bought over the counter and it has remarkable properties. It is a Qi tonic and is used in strengthening Qi depleted by long illness, ageing or stress. In TCM terms, it nourishes Yang of Spleen and Lung, aids upward circulation of Qi, improves Protective Qi, and calms the mind. It is very strong and quite hot in its nature. Prolonged use actually depletes the Qi.

A client came for hot rashes appearing on his jawline, down his body and the front of the legs. After questioning about diet, lifestyle and other problems, he told me that he took ginseng every day to help his energy because he exercised every day for up to four hours. The combination of the Heat from the exercise and the ginseng caused the Heat to vent through the skin. After a week without ginseng, his rash had eased greatly. A month later there was no trace, and he also had more energy. Menopausal women who experience hot flushes should not take ginseng on its own because its warm nature plus its ability to aid upward circulation of Qi usually makes the problem worse.

Dang Gui

Known as angelica in the West, this herb has recently been discovered by some Western practitioners as a woman's herb. It is certainly used mainly in gynaecological formulas and Blood problems. Its nature is warm and it activates Blood circulation. In TCM terms, it nourishes the Blood, moistens the intestines, regulates the female reproductive system, and detoxifies Blood. Since it is a Blood-moving herb, it needs to be taken with respect. Although it is used in formulas during pregnancy, if there is a deficiency during this time it should not be used. I also feel that, if it is taken on its own for a Blood deficiency, it may aggravate this condition.

Astragalus or Huang Qi

This is a herb that is used in the treatment of severe Qi deficiency. It appears to have a stimulating effect on the immune system and is being used in the treatment of people infected with AIDS and HIV. It has also been used to treat the side-effects of cancer therapies. In TCM terms, it strengthens Protective Qi, aids upward circulation of Qi, strengthens Spleen, and assists in tonifying Yin. This herb is safe to use in large doses and can be added to soups as a good Qi tonic.

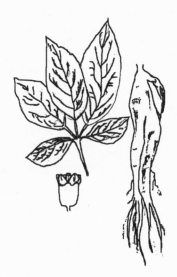

Figure 19. Ginseng.

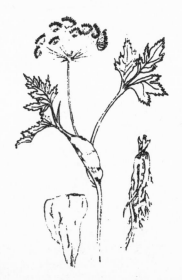

Figure 20. Dang gui or angelica.

Cornsilk

This is a safe herb that can be used as a tea to alleviate the effects of UTI. Cornsilk is sweet and neutral, and affects Liver, Gall Bladder and Urinary Bladder. In TCM terms, it is diuretic, anti-hypertensive and haemostatic, and reduces blood sugar.

Ginger

As a tea, ginger calms rebellious Stomach Qi, so it is useful for nausea, especially morning sickness. As a poultice (fresh ginger grated and applied) it is very warming and can help Cold-affected arthritis. Applied to the abdomen, it relieves period pain. In TCM terms, it is pungent and warm, affecting the Lung, Stomach and Spleen. It is a diaphoretic (promotes perspiration), an anti-emetic (relieves nausea) and an expectorant. It should not be used where there are Heat signs, especially due to Yin deficiency.

Peppermint

As a tea, it calms nausea and relieves colic pain. It is pungent and cool, affecting the Lung and Liver. In TCM terms, it dispels Wind and Heat, clears the head and eyes, and relieves stagnant Liver Qi.

Raspberry Leaf

Tea made from raspberry leaf is helpful in childbirth. It causes the muscles of the uterus to contract. It should not be used in the first trimester, especially by women prone to habitual miscarriage. Raspberry fruit or *fu pen zi* has a different effect. It is sweet, sour and

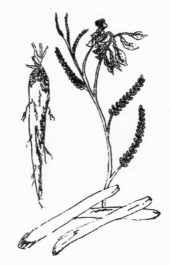

Figure 21. Astragalus or huang qi.

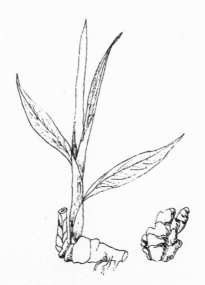

Figure 22. Ginger.

slightly warm, and it affects Liver and Kidney. In TCM terms, it tonifies the Liver and Kidney, astringes urine and semen, and brightens the eyes. It is a useful herb in combination for sterility or infertility because of its association with Kidney.

Diet

Diet is a form of therapy and important in support of a TCM treatment to continue good health. The basis of Chinese dietary therapy is that energy is needed to make Blood from the food ingested.

Think of the stomach as a large pot of boiling water; if you add raw, cold vegetables to this pot, the water stops boiling. The pot now needs to be bought back to the boil by using more heat (energy). If the digestive fire is low or unsatisfactory, adding cold and raw foods will further deplete it. More energy is needed to break down (digest) the food. When energy is low, food is not completely broken down. Undigested food may be passed through the bowel, but sometimes it remains in the body and adds to a Damp or Phlegm condition. If food is not digested correctly, the body is unable to extract enough nutrients to form Blood and Qi. This is why soups are so nutritious and useful as a remedial diet when Qi and Blood are deficient.

In TCM, the Stomach breaks down food in a situation similar to the boiling pot, creating food essences. This food essence is moved (transported) and changed (transformed) by Spleen. Spleen absorbs the nourishment from food, separating the usable from the unusable. Spleen is the primary organ in the production of Qi. Food Qi of the Spleen is also the basis for the formation of Blood. Spleen does important work and needs its energy for other areas. It is best if it is not impeded by raw and cold foods or irregular eating patterns.

The main aspects of TCM dietary therapy are to take small amounts of cold or uncooked foods; to avoid cold (refrigerated) water and other drinks; and to reduce the intake of coffee and alcohol. Eat warm foods in winter, cool foods in summer. All foods have a nature, whether cold, warm or neutral, and a knowledge of these foods in relation to yourself and your environment is useful. For further reading on the nature of foods, refer to Appendix 5.

I do not believe it is necessary to be highly regimented in your diet: rather, moderation is the key. If you really need coffee in the morning to get going, go ahead and have it; if you deny yourself the coffee, you raise your stress level, both emotional and physical. However, if you habitually drink three or more cups of coffee a day, it is kinder to yourself to reduce the amount slowly. Coffee's nature is Cold (this does not refer to caffeine content, so decaffeinated coffee is also Cold). Cold restricts Blood flow; when pain is present, reduced Blood flow contributes to stronger pain. There are some writers who see coffee as having a warm, energetic nature. If they are correct, resulting effects in regard to pain still hold: warmth can congeal Damp into Phlegm, causing blockage and ultimately pain.

To reduce coffee intake, two strategies seem to work:

- Every second cup, forget to add the coffee to the warm water and drink this water slowly.
- Create a special ritual with coffee. Sit down, prepare a time and space, and relish the specialness of this *one cup of beautiful coffee*.

The current fashion for taking plenty of raw foods and cold drinks in order to reduce weight is in opposition to TCM. If you lead a very active life with a large amount of physical exercise (for instance, full training for the Olympic Games), then raw foods and cold drinks are not such a problem. The high level of physical exercise creates Heat (Yang) in the body and so it has the energy to break down the undigested food. The problem occurs in a sedentary or low-exercise lifestyle. There is less Yang to burn up or metabolise raw foods, which can possibly lead to retention of undigested food in your system. This undigested food, over a period of time, can manifest such problems as lethargy, weight gain, fluid retention, digestive and bowel problems, lowered immune response, and general weakness.

To have warm foods does not mean lots of chilli or curries. More appropriate are cooked foods without spices, preferably served warm. Soups are an excellent food to help your digestion to respond. Steaming or stir-frying are other ways of preparing warm and digested food. If you enjoy salad, you can support your digestive system by giving it a kickstart with a cup of clear soup to warm the stomach, about 10 minutes before you eat the salad.

I have often been asked about my feelings towards a macrobiotic diet. It can be healthy and balanced if correctly applied, although it is alien to most Australian tastes. It can also be seen as highly regimented method of eating which does not allow for the variances in our lives, such as eating out or at friends' homes. Part of the philosophy of macrobiotics is similar to Chinese dietary therapy, where a balance of Yin and Yang is needed. The other part is to eat food that is grown locally, is not overprocessed, and is seasonally appropriate. A pineapple eaten in winter in Melbourne is opposed to this thought. The pineapple is not locally grown (it comes from Queensland) and is not seasonally correct (it is a summer fruit). This philosophy is easily followed, even with an Australian diet of many varied styles.

Suggested foods for particular conditions are given below, and soup recipes are provided in Appendix 2. For more extensive food lists and recipes, refer to the books listed in Appendix 5.

Foods to Avoid:
- *Heat*: alcohol, spicy and fried foods.
- *Pain*: cold and sour foods, coffee.
- *Oedema* (Fluid Retention): shellfish.
- *Asthma*: cold and raw foods.
- *Stomach and intestinal problems*: steak, roast beef, sour and cold foods.
- *Congestion and mucous*: bananas, milk.
- *Uro-genital*: yeast foods (bread, beer, wine).

Foods for Blood Deficiency

Liver, leafy green vegetables, grapes, lamb, beef, pumpkin, pork, miso, abalone, Chinese red dates, anchovy, kidney beans, beetroot, chicken, coconut, fig.

Foods for Liver Qi

Beef and chicken livers (pâté), black sesame, celery, mussels, plum, bay leaf, basil, beetroot, black pepper, cabbage, coconut milk, garlic, ginger, leek, marjoram, rosemary, saffron, spring onions, peach. Take the warmer-natured foods (such as ginger, marjoram, black pepper) with caution if there are Liver Heat signs.

Avoid: Alcohol, coffee, deep-fried greasy foods, spices, red meat, sugar, chemicals, drugs, tobacco, marijuana.

Foods for Cold Damp

Barley, corn, adzuki beans, pumpkin, mustard greens, daikon, turnip, sourdough, garlic, alfalfa, tuna, chicken, celery.

Avoid: Milk and products, cheese, sugar, shellfish, eggs, wheat, fruit, cucumber, soya beans, spinach, olives, olive oil, pork.

Foods for Hot Damp

As for Cold Damp, plus *Lactobacillus* in powder or pill form (not in yoghurt because it is a dairy product and contraindicated).

Avoid: Alcohol, coffee, tea, dairy foods, sugar, fruits, fatty foods, spices, garlic, pork, red meat, shellfish, yeast foods, wheat, refined food, chemicals.

Foods for Cold

Pumpkin, carrot, sweet potato, leek, rice, oats, congee (rice porridge), chicken, turkey, ginger; warm fluids only.

Avoid: Salads, citrus fruits, juices, excess salt, tofu (unless marinated and dry baked), milk, cheese, excess liquids, excess sweet foods.

Final Note

By now you will have realised that raw, cold and refrigerated foods are not the best for maintenance of health. This does not mean that you cannot have these foods, but moderation is the key.

Balance and moderation of diet and lifestyle, making adjustments as needed depending on climate, stress factors and emotions, will help to keep you healthy. Forewarned is forearmed.

The idea of this book is to arm you with information that will help you understand your body in TCM terms. The main thing to remember is moderation. Of course you can have salads, moderately; yes, you can have an alcoholic drink in moderation; sure, have a coffee, but be moderate in your consumption.

Balance and moderation are the key words.

Appendixes

1. Moxabustion

Moxabustion (moxa) is a common treatment in TCM and is used particularly in winter. Moxa is a method of applying localised heat to points of certain parts of the body.

Moxa material is a herb, *Artemisia vulgaris*, a chrysanthemum. To quote a Chinese scholar:

> The moxa leaf is bitter, acrid, producing warmth when used in small amounts and strong heat when used in large amounts. It is of pure Yang nature . . . It can open the 12 regular meridians, travelling through the three Yin meridians to regulate Qi and Blood, expel cold and dampness, warm the uterus, stop bleeding, warm the spleen and stomach to remove stagnation, regulate menstruation and ease the foetus . . . When burned, it penetrates all the meridians.[*]

The function of moxa is to warm the meridians and

---

[*]Cheng Xinnong, (1990) *Chinese Acupuncture and Moxibustion*, p. 340.

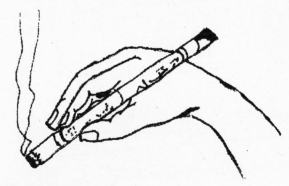

Figure 23. The correct way to hold a moxa stick.

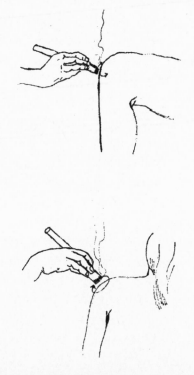

Figure 24. The moxa stick is used to warm the meridians and expel Cold.

expel Cold, and to induce the smooth flow of Qi and Blood. Moxa strengthens Yang from collapsing, and it also prevents disease to keep the body healthy.

Moxa comes in the form of cigar-like sticks or cones, or loose (punk). Moxa sticks are held directly over a point or meridian. Moxa cones are placed on slices of ginger or garlic, which are then placed over points. Punk is used in boxes, which are placed on broad flat areas; punk is also used on needles.

To use a moxa stick, it is easiest to light it with a candle. It can take a little while to ignite evenly and a candle is a safe method. Gently blow on the burning end of the stick to get a strong even glow. Hold the lit stick directly over a selected meridian point, about 3–5 cm above (do not place moxa directly onto the skin). Hold it there for 5–10 minutes, until the area is glowing red or feels hot. Move the stick around the area and return to the point, till it once more warms up. A moxa stick can also be moved along a meridian: hold the stick a little away from the surface of the skin (3–5 cm) and move the stick along the affected area.

To extinguish the moxa stick, either stand it up in a bowl of uncooked rice (do not push or grind into rice), or mould a square of tinfoil on the ignited end to extinguish it.

I suggest that moxa not be used until you have consulted your TCM practitioner to make sure that it is the correct treatment for your condition and that you understand the methods.

2. Soup Recipes

Soups help to build Blood and support Spleen and Stomach functions. They are quick and easy to prepare and easily digested. Soups are the easiest way to have warm and well-digested food. These recipes yield approximately four servings, depending whether they are for a meal (2–3) or entree (4–5).

Vegetable Broth
To calm Liver Yang and support Spleen.

2 cloves garlic, chopped	3 tomatoes (fresh or tinned)
2 onions	1 slice ginger
3 carrots	6 strands saffron (optional)
2 sticks celery	½ cup barley (optional)
1 parsnip	pepper and salt
½ small turnip	2 tablespoons soya sauce
½ small swede	1 tablespoon vegetable oil

Chop vegetables. In a pan, sauté garlic and onions with ½ teaspoon sugar till brown. Remove onions. In remaining oil, brown carrots, celery, parsnip, turnip and swede.

Place all of the above ingredients in a soup pot.

Cover with water, and add tomatoes, ginger, saffron, and seasoning (barley). Bring to the boil, and simmer for 45 minutes.

Lamb Shank Broth
To tonify Spleen and Kidney.

1 cup barley
3 lamb shanks
2 sticks of celery
1 large onion
1 parsnip

2 cloves garlic
2 carrots
1 tablespoon soya sauce
pepper and salt

Soak barley overnight. Chop vegetables. Cover shanks and vegetables with water, and add 2 cups water. Add seasoning. Bring to the boil.

When simmering, add barley. Simmer for two hours. Remove shanks, take meat from shanks, chop small and return to the soup.

Because of the fat content of lamb it is best to leave it to stand overnight in the refrigerator to allow the fat to congeal. The fat can then be lifted off and discarded.

Serve warm with crusty bread, preferably sourdough; or with shell pasta, rice or egg noodles.

For a variation, omit the lamb shanks and replace the water with chicken or beef stock.

Bean and Bacon Soup
To move Liver stagnation.

1 large onion
½ teaspoon sugar
3 cloves garlic, chopped
3 rashers bacon, chopped
½ capsicum
2 sticks celery
2 carrots
2 tomatoes, thinly sliced
4 cups chicken or beef
   stock

large tin three-bean mix
(or 2 cups mixed beans—
   bortolli, kidney, etc.—
   soaked overnight and
   cooked for 1 hour)
1 cup uncooked pasta
   shells
pepper and salt
parmesan cheese

In a small amount of olive oil or sesame oil, cook chopped onion with sugar till brown. Add garlic and bacon.

Chop vegetables, and place in a pot with bacon and onion mixture. Add either chicken stock (lighter flavour) or beef stock. Add beans, bring to the boil, simmer 20 minutes.

Add pasta and simmer another 10 minutes till pasta is cooked.

Serve with croutons, sprinkled with grated parmesan cheese.

Chinese Combination Soup
To build blood, calm Liver and support Spleen.

thin noodles

chicken stock made with
ginger and garlic

8 wantons (steamed, not
fried)

150 g Chinese red pork,
thinly sliced

chicken breast, thinly
sliced

100 g firm bean curd
(tofu), sliced thinly

8 green prawns

12 snow peas or 4 leaves of
bok choy, sliced

6 spring onions, chopped
finely

pepper and salt

Cook noodles and put aside.

Bring chicken stock to the boil. Add wantons, pork, chicken, bean curd, prawns and then bok choy or snow peas. Simmer 7 minutes till cooked, take off the heat.

In each bowl place some cooked noodles and spring onions. Pour the stock mixture over the noodles. Try to even out the contents between bowls.

Pea and Ham Soup
To build Blood.

500 g split green peas or
lentils

1 ham hock

1 large onion, chopped

1 tablespoon spice balls

3 bay leaves

pepper (no salt needs to
be added because of the
ham hock)

Simmer split peas for 1 hour, (peas can be cooked in a microwave oven for 15 minutes). Drain off the water.

In a large soup pot, place ham hock, cooked peas, onion and spices. Cover with water, and add 2 cups of water. Bring to the boil, simmer 2 hours. Every 20 minutes or so, scoop the bubbles from the top, and then stir the soup to prevent the peas from sticking to the pot.

Remove hock, cut away meat, put aside. Let soup stand overnight, scrape off fat.

Soup consistency should be very thick, almost able to be cut with a knife. On heating, this will soften. Add chicken stock to dilute soup to your requirements.

Serve soup with the chopped meat from the hock.

Chicken Soup

To build Blood, strengthen Lung Qi, move Phlegm and support Spleen.

1 chicken (No. 4) or 1 kg chicken necks and bones	slice ginger (thumbnail size)
1 large onion	2 cloves garlic, chopped
½ capsicum, sliced thinly	4–6 strands saffron
2 carrots	1 tablespoon soya sauce
1 stick celery	pepper and salt

Chop the vegetables and joint the chicken. Put all ingredients in a pot. Cover with water and bring to the boil. Simmer for 1 hour for a roasting chicken, 2 hours for bones or a boiler. When cooked, remove chicken or bones and let soup stand overnight in the fridge.

Next day remove most of the fat that has congealed on the top. Leave a little in the soup for flavour. Serve with egg noodles and chopped spring onions, or with rice or matzo balls.

Matzo Balls

2 cups matzo meal (or
   crushed matzo)
1 egg
1 tablespoon water

1 tablespoon oil
pepper and salt
clear chicken stock

Mix all ingredients except stock and let stand 1 hour. Roll tablespoonfuls into balls. Cook for approximately 7 minutes in stock till floating and firm.

When cooked, remove from stock. If serving with chicken soup, add matzo balls when heating to serve.

Mushroom Abalone Soup
To cool rising Liver Yang, clear heat in Lung.

1 tablespoon sesame oil
3 spring onions, chopped
2 cloves garlic
1 slice of ginger
6 dried mushrooms
1 teaspoon soya sauce
½ teaspoon sugar

1 abalone fillet, thinly
   sliced
½ cup snow peas
1 tablespoon cornflour
   dissolved in 3 cups
   water

Soak mushrooms in water for one hour, remove stems and slice thinly.

Heat oil in a wok. Add spring onions, garlic, ginger and mushrooms, together with sugar and soya sauce, and brown quickly. Add the abalone and peas, stir for 1 minute. Add water and cornflour mixture, and stir till the soup thickens slightly. Serve as an appetiser.

Chinese Tomato Soup
To lower and cool rising Liver Yang.

1 large tomato, cut in wedges	bacon
1 large onion, cut in wedges	4 cups hot water
3½ tablespoons vegetable oil	1 chicken stock cube (without MSG)
2 tablespoons chopped	salt
	1 egg

Heat oil in wok and sauté the onions, tomato and bacon. Add hot water and stock cube, bring to the boil. Simmer for 5 minutes.

Season with salt. Stir in beaten egg little by little, quickly over a high heat. Serve.

Ox Tail Soup
To build Blood, Spleen and Stomach.

1 kg oxtails	2 carrots
½ teaspoon sugar	1 large onion
½ teaspoon ginger powder	1 parsnip
2 cloves garlic	3 sticks celery
1 turnip	½ cup barley
½ swede	½ teaspoon mixed herbs

Chop vegetables and place all the ingredients in a large pot. Cover with water and cook for 2½ to 3 hours till meat is soft on the bone. Remove the bones, take all the meat from them and return it to the soup.

Leave the soup overnight in the refrigerator to allow the fat to congeal so it can be scraped off.

Serve with pasta or macaroni.

Chicken or Beef Stock

chicken or chopped beef marrow bones	pepper and salt
saffron	1 tablespoon soya sauce
garlic	1 onion, chopped

Cover all ingredients with water. Bring to the boil and simmer for at least 1 hour, 2 hours if beef bones are used. Strain liquid, stand overnight in refrigerator, and remove fat. Quantities can be frozen till needed.

3. Medicated Liqueurs and Tinctures

Liqueurs are useful, especially during autumn and winter, for specific needs such as coughs, cold or headaches.

Liqueurs are herbs soaked in alcohol for a period of one month. Alcohol is the prime ingredient and its nature is warm, sweet, pungent and ascending. It enters the Lung, Stomach, Heart and Liver meridians. Alcohol assists Yang, and tonifies Qi and Blood. Alcohol also regulates the Qi, expels Cold, removes Blood stagnation, opens up the meridians, facilitates circulation, and reinforces the action of the herbs combined with it.

A little alcohol is a valuable medicine. It is used, in moderation, in deficiency conditions characterised by Cold or reduced circulation.

Excessive use of alcohol harms the stomach, causing it to become Hot, and depletes the Stomach Yin. It harms Liver and Heart and causes Damp to accumulate. Alcohol is dispersing and if taken in large amounts can make the body susceptible to external pathogenic invasion.

Vodka is the most neutral form of alcohol available and is appropriate for these tinctures.

For Headache

30 g walnut kernels   50 ml vodka
50 g white sugar

Grind walnuts till fine, mix with sugar. Add vodka and simmer for 10 minutes.

Take a teaspoonful twice daily with a glass of warm water.

This tincture tonifies Lungs and Kidneys, transforms sputum, relieves cough.

For Influenza Headache

100 g sunflower seeds   vodka to cover
100 g sunflower leaf

Soak for 12 hours, strain and store.

Take 1 teaspoonful in half a glass of warm water, three times a day.

For Common Cold with Headache and Mild Fever

60 g chrysanthemums   200 ml vodka
60 g wolfberry (*gou qi zi*)   20 g honey

Soak flowers and berries in alcohol for 10–20 days. Then stir in honey and store.

Take 1 teaspoonful twice a day

For Cough or Indigestion

30 g tangerine or mandarin   500 ml vodka
   peel

Soak peel in alcohol for 7 days, shaking regularly. Strain and discard peel.

Take 1 tablespoonful before sleep.

For Indigestion, Regurgitation of Food From Stomach

10 g cardamom, crushed   250 ml rice wine
5 g hawthorn fruit
   (*shan zha*)

Soak for 7–10 days. Strain and discard solids.
   Take 1 teaspoonful twice a day with a glass of warm water.

For Vomiting

5 ml ginger juice   20 ml grape wine (no
                                preservative)

Combine ingredients, shake well.
   Sip 1 tablespoon twice a day.

4. Shopping List

Fu ling, *Poria cocos* (fungus)
Hong zao, Chinese red date
Gou qi zi, wolfberry
Huang qi, astragalus
Adzuki beans
Chrysanthemum flowers
Qing pe, tangerine peel
Sha ren, cardamom
Shan zha, hawthorn fruit
Tao ren, walnut kernels
Mi ren, Chinese barley
Umeboshi plums

Patent Formulas
   Yin Chiao
   Gan Mao Ling
   Watermelon Frost
   Tiger Balm

Most of these herbs and pills are available from Chinese grocery stores. Chinese medicine practitioners can supply the patent formulas.

5. Suggested Reading

There are many books on TCM available: the following is a list of those I have found to be of particular use.

Traditional Chinese Medicine

Beinfold, Harriet and Efrem Korngold, *Between Heaven and Earth*, Ballantine Books, 1991.

Hoizey, Dominique, and Marie-Joseph Hoizey, *A History of Chinese Medicine*, Edinburgh University Press, 1988.

Kaptchuk, Fred J., *The Web that Has No Weaver*, Congdon and Weed Inc., 1983.

Diet

Beinfold, Harriet, and Efrem Korngold, *Between Heaven and Earth*, Ballantine Books, 1991.

Flaws, Bob, *Arisal of the Clear*, Blue Poppy Press, 1991.

Flaws, Bob, and Honora Wolfe, *Prince Wen Hui's Cook*, Paradigm Press, 1983.

Lu, Henry C., *Chinese System of Food Cures*, Sterling Publishing Co., 1986.

Wilson, Geoffrey D., *Take this Pebble From my Hand*, Seventh Heaven Books, 1993.

Stress Management

Gach, Michael Reed, and Carolyn Marco, *Acu-Yoga*,
    Japan Publications Inc., 1981.

References

ACMERC (Australian Chinese Medicine Education and Research Council), *Newsletter*, Vol 1, 2 November 1995.

Beinfeld, Harriet and Efrem Korngold, *Between Heaven and Earth*, Ballantine Books, USA, 1991.

Cathay Herbal Labs, *Newsletter*, Summer 1996.

Flaws, Bob, *Arisal of the Clear*, Blue Poppy Press, USA, 1991.

Flaws, Bob, *Something Old, Something New*, Blue Poppy Press, USA, 1991.

Flaws, Bob, *Free and Easy*, Blue Poppy Press, USA, 1990.

Flaws, Bob, and Honora Wolfe, *Prince Wen Hui's Cook*, Paradigm Press, USA, 1983.

Friedan, Betty, *The Foundation of Age*, Jonathon Cape, London, 1993.

Hammer, Leon, *Dragon Rises Red Bird Flies*, Crucible, Thorsons Publishing, UK, 1990.

Hoizey, Dominique and Mare-Joseph Hoizey, *A History of Chinese Medicine*, Edinburgh University Press, 1988.

Hsu, Hong-Yen & Su-Yen Wang, *The Theory of Feverish Diseases and its Clinical Applications*,

Oriental Healing Arts Institute, USA, 1985.

Jiayi, Liu & Liu Peilu & Sun Yingjie, *Diagnostics of Traditional Chinese* Medicine, Publishing House of Shanghai College of TCM, 1990.

Kaptchuk, Ted, *The Web that Has No Weaver*, Congdon & Weed, USA, 1983.

Li, Shih-Chen, *Pulse Diagnosis*, Paradigm Press, USA, 1985.

Lu, Henry C., *Chinese System of Food Cures*, Sterling Publishing Co, USA, 1986.

Maciocia, Giovanni, *The Foundations of Chinese Medicine*, Churchill Livingstone, UK, 1995.

Maciocia, Giovanni, *The Practice of Chinese Medicine* Churchill Livingstone, UK, 1995.

Maciocia, Giovanni, *Tongue Diagnosis in Chinese Medicine*, Eastland Press, USA, 1987.

Nong,Sang, *Chinese Medicated Liquor Therapy*, Beijing Science and Technology Press, 1996.

Ross, Jeremy, and Zang Fu, *The Organ System of Traditional Chinese Medicine*, 2nd ed., Churchill Livingstone, UK, 1989.

Wilson, Geoffrey D., *Take this Pebble From My Hand*, Seventh Heaven Publishing, Australia, 1993.

Wolfe, Honora, *Second Spring*, Blue Poppy Press, USA, 1990.

Worwood, Valerie Ann, *The Fragrant Pharmacy*, Bantam Books, 1990.

Xinnong, Cheng, *Chinese Acupuncture and Moxibustion*, Foreign Language Press, China, 1990.

INDEX